AN INTRODUCTION TO
EAR DISEASE

AN INTRODUCTION TO
EAR DISEASE

Bruce Black

F.R.A.C.S., F.R.C.S. (Ed.), F.R.C.S.
Clinical Professor, Otolaryngology
University of Queensland

Chairman
Department of Otolaryngology
Royal Children's Hospital

Audiological sections in conjunction with

David Brown-Rothwell, M.Sc.(Psych), M.Sc.(Aud)

Singular Publishing Group, Inc.
San Diego · London

MW

Singular Publishing Group, Inc.
401 West "A" Street, Suite 325
San Diego, California 92101-7904

Singular Publishing Ltd.
19 Compton Terrace
London, N1 2UN, UK

Singular Publishing Group, Inc., publishes textbooks, clinical manuals, clinical reference books, journals, videos, and multimedia materials on speech-language pathology, audiology, otorhinolaryngology, special education, early childhood, aging, occupational therapy, physical therapy, rehabilitation, counseling, mental health, and voice. For your convenience, our entire catalog can be accessed on our website at *http://www.singpub.com*. Our mission to provide you with materials to meet the daily challenges of the ever-changing health care/educational environment will remain on course if we are in touch with you. In that spirit, we welcome your feedback on our products. Please telephone (**1-800-521-8545**), fax (**1-800-774-8398**), or e-mail (*singpub@mail.cerfnet.com*) your comments and requests to us.

© 1999 by Singular Publishing Group, Inc.

Printed in the United States of America by BookCrafters

Library of Congress Cataloging-in-Publication Data

Black, Bruce, F.R.A.C.S.
    Introduction to ear disease / Bruce Black : audiological sections
in conjunction with David Brown-Rothwell.
        p.   cm.
    ISBN 0-7693-0012-X
    1. Ear—Diseases.   I. Brown-Rothwell, David.   II. Title.
    [DNLM: 1. Ear Diseases.   WV 200B6271 1998]
RF121.B53   1998
617.8'9—dc21
DNLM/DLC
for Library of Congress   98–36570
                                                               CIP

11/21/02

CONTENTS

INTRODUCTION

This work has been 20 years in evolution. Clinical experience in otology during that time often required close interaction with family physicians and medical students and this demonstrated the need for a hands-on, do-it-yourself ready reference work, amply illustrated and with a maximal "must know" and "should know" content. Prior to this work, the literature has lacked a specialized comprehensive ear text at a basic level. Previous works were either color atlases or general otorhinolaryngological works, but each lacked the combined photographic, line illustration, and lecture note-type text herein, specialized solely into ear disease.

The work is intended for professionals who seek solutions for everyday ear problems. These include family physicians, medical students, junior otolaryngology residents, accident and emergency staff, specialized nurses; and audiologists, among others. Probably, there are many such personnel who, when confronted with an otological problem which may be difficult to diagnose and treat, will find the text of some help, and to them the work is dedicated.

I would like to thank my staff who, over the years, have typed, photocopied, revised, and reworked the project during its prolonged gestation. In particular, my thanks to to Jane, Mary, Michelle, Ali, and Chrissie. Also, I would like to thank SmithKline Beecham for their support in an earlier promotional publication. Lastly, I wish to thank the staff of Singular Publishing Group, particularly for their impressive efficiency in rapidly implementing publication.

Bruce Black
Fig Tree Pocket, Brisbane, 1998

To Janie and Jenny,
Remarkable ladies, both.

CHAPTER 1:
UNDERSTANDING THE EAR

The ear is a series of three compartments, the external, middle and inner ears. (Fig. 1) Fortunately diseases of the ear usually afflict one compartment at a time. Therefore to understand the presentation of disease, one requires an understanding of each compartment's normal anatomy and function.

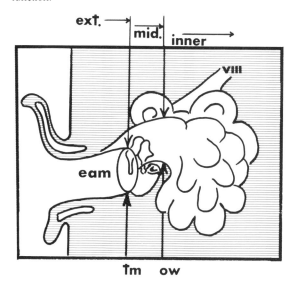

Figure 1.   Compartments of the ear. Anatomically, the ear divides into external, middle and inner divisions. As a rule, disease tends to affect only one compartment at a time. This helps the clinician considerably during diagnosis of ear pathology. tm: tympanic membrane; ow: oval window; eam: external auditory meatus.

1. ANATOMY AND PHYSIOLOGY

1.1 EXTERNAL EAR

The pinna and external canal are similar to a hearing horn. In man, the pinna has only rudimentary sound gathering purposes and is largely expendable. The external canal, by contrast, has three functions:

(a) Sound Conduction:
> The external canal permits sound to reach the ear drum and ossicular chain. Total obstruction of the canal, as in congenital atresia, produces deafness as severe as 70–80 decibels. If the canal is blocked by debris, hearing is lost appreciably only when total canal occlusion occurs. A small chink between obstructing exostoses or around a mass of wax may render the blockage asymptomatic.

(b) Defence of the tympanic membrane:
> (i) S Curve. The entrance to the external canal is guarded by an overlap of the conchal bowl cartilage. The canal itself is curved, sometimes markedly so. These factors combine to prevent direct, penetrating injuries.

> (ii) Sensitivity. The canal is progressively highly sensitive towards the tympanic membrane. This helps avoid self injury.

> (iii) Cerumen. The canal "wax" discourages intrusion by insects and helps collect dust for expulsion.

(c) Self Cleaning:
> The squamous epithelium of the canal constantly migrates towards the exterior, originating from the tympanic membrane. The migration carries dust and wax laterally, preventing "silting up" of the deep canal.

Principal structures:

(a) Tympanic membrane

(b) Ossicular chain

(c) Eustachian tube

(a) Tympanic membrane

The drum has a shape similar to the shallow, curved cone structure of a loud speaker, with the centre at the tip of the handle of the malleus. Due to the angulation of the external meatus, the malleus appears to pass posteroinferiorly on external inspection. The cone shape provides optimal acoustic pick–up. The tympanic membrane is normally taut and transparent, but becomes slightly sclerosed or "milky" with age.

(b) Ossicular chain

The three ossicles (malleus, incus and stapes) function as a lever system (malleus and incus) which rotates to drive a piston (stapes). The malleus handle is 1.3 times as long as the incus (Fig. 2) and the total area of the tympanic membrane is approximately twenty times the area of the stapes footplate (Fig. 3). These two factors combine to enhance sound transmission through the middle ear and footplate to the cochlea.

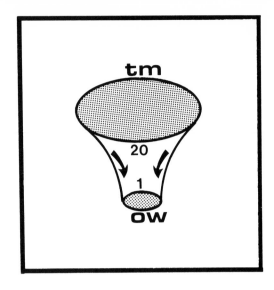

Figure 3.   Relative sizes of the tympanic membrane and the oval window. The middle ear mechanisms concentrate the sound from the tympanic membrane on to the oval window. tm: tympanic membrane; ow: oval window.

(c) Eustachian tube

The eustachian tube is the "trachea" of the ear. Its prime function is to equalise pressure inside and outside the tympanic membrane such that the latter is not under undue pressure, and therefore strain. In addition, whilst the middle ear is air–containing, the ossicular chain can vibrate freely with minimal hindrance. The tube is normally closed to seal off the ear from pressure changes during respiration and to prevent autophony. It is actively opened by the tensor palati during swallowing, yawning or other palate manoeuvres. The tensor palati, which hooks around the pterygoid hamulus in a pulley effect, meets its partner in the midline raphe of the soft palate. This provides anchorage inferiorly, whilst the muscle pulls down on the tubal cartilage to open the tube itself. At the same time, the soft palate is pulled superiorly, thus closing the nasopharynx to protect the nose from spillover as it opens the eustachian tube. (Fig. 4)

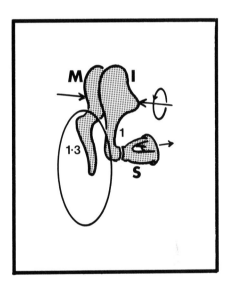

Figure 2.   Middle ear ossicular mechanisms. The ossicles form a lever system and a piston system. The malleus and incus function as a unit, rotating on an axis between the anterior malleolar ligament and the short process of the incus. The shorter incus thus permits greater mechanical leverage on the piston formed by the stapes. M: malleus; I: incus; S: stapes.

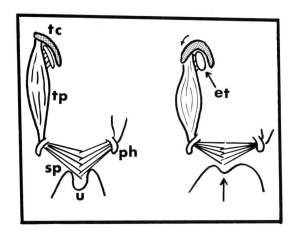

Figure 4.   Musculature of the palate and eustachian tube. The eustachian tube is normally closed and applied close to the tubal cartilage. The latter is pulled into a U–shape by the tensor palati. The change in shape of the cartilage induces tubal opening. tc: tubal cartilage; tp: tensor palati; sp: soft palate; u: uvula; ph: pterygoid hamulus; et: eustachian tube.

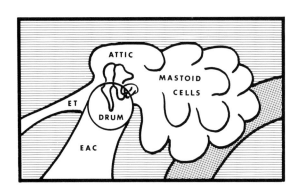

Figure 5.   Plan of the middle ear cleft. Air enters via the eustachian tube, passes through the middle ear, attic and aditus and is absorbed via the mastoid air cell system. ET: eustachian tube; EAC: external auditory canal.

Upon opening of the tube, air passes to the middle ear cleft and is subsequently absorbed into the mucosa of the middle ear cleft and mastoid air cell system. (Fig. 5) There is thus a dynamic replacement of the middle ear air. Failure of this function results in many of the major middle ear diseases. The precise role of the mastoid air cell system remains uncertain. It probably acts as a buffer against rapid pressure changes which would otherwise produce tension on the drum.

1.3 INNER EAR

Principle structures:

(a) Cochlea

(b) Vestibular Apparatus

(a) Cochlea.

The "snailshell" of the cochlea contains the array of sound receptor cells. Cells at the basal end receive the

higher frequencies (8000 cps), those at the apex, the lower tones (250 cps). The cochlea is a combined transducer and computer terminal. Sound (kinetic energy) vibrates the tectorial membrane causing distortion of the filaments of the hair cells of the organ of Corti. Distortion of the filaments induces action potentials (electrical energy). These potentials are then coded and relayed via the acoustic nerve (VIII) to the central computer, the brain. (Fig. 6)

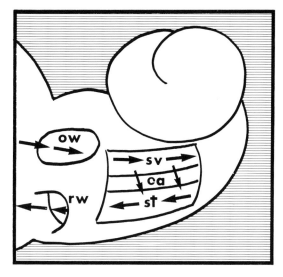

Figure 6.   Passage of sound through the cochlea. Sound enters via the oval window, passes up the scala vestibuli and across the cochlea aqueduct. It then leaves via the scala tympani and exits through the round window. ow: oval window; rw: round window; sv: scala vestibuli; ca: cochlear aqueduct; st: scala tympani.

(b) Vestibular Apparatus.

The vestibular balance mechanisms incorporate hair cell organs with an overlying body of jelly–like tissue containing calcite otoliths. The cellular function of the balance mechanism is similar to the cochlea. Physical forces cause the movement of the cupula or statoconial membrane relative to the filaments of the vestibular sensory cells. Distortion of the filament produces action potentials which are then passed to the central nervous system via the vestibular branch of the eighth nerve. The vestibular apparatus is divided into the utricle and saccule, and the lateral semi–circular canals. The two areas have different functions:

(i) Utricle and saccule: Detection of gravity, perception of acceleration and deceleration.

(ii) Semi–circular canals: Detection of rotary movement (Fig. 7)

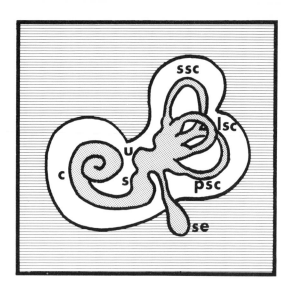

Figure 7.   The membranous labyrinth. c: cochlear spiral; s: saccule; u: utricle; ssc: superior semicircular canal; lsc: lateral semicircular canal; psc: posterior semicircular canal; se: saccus endolymphaticus.

2. ASSESSMENT OF EAR DISEASE

2.1 HISTORY

2.2 PHYSICAL EXAMINATION

2.3 EXAMINATION OF HEARING

2.4 AUDIOMETRY

2.5 OTHER INVESTIGATIONS

2.1 HISTORY

Disease in each compartment of the ear presents with one or more cardinal symptoms:

(a) Pain
(b) Discharge } Common in infection or inflammation.

(c) Deafness
(d) Tinnitus } Aberrations of hearing i.e. too little sound or abnormal sound is reported.

(e) Vertigo   Vestibular aberrations present as hallucinations of movement.

A sixth symptom, cranial nerve palsies, may also be present. Facial nerve palsy is the most common.

A thorough interrogation of each symptom must be made along the usual lines, i.e.
(a) Site
(b) Nature
(c) Severity
(d) Duration
(e) Onset
(f) Aggravating or relieving factors
(g) Associated factors

(h) Radiation (pain)

Each symptom may give strong clues as to the nature of the disease process:

(a) Pain

Enquire as to the precise location of the pain, particularly pain in or near the ear, e.g. in the temporomandibular joint. Pain in the ear is covered in depth in the chapter on Otalgia.

(b) Discharge

The nature of discharge will suggest its origin:

(i) A watery discharge, particularly in the presence of pruritis, often indicates an external origin, particularly after scratching.

(ii) Mucus in the discharge indicates a middle ear origin as there are no goblet cells in the external canal.

(iii) A foul odour associated with the discharge usually means a chronic middle ear origin.

(iv) Bleeding may be from trauma, a granulation or a vascular ear tumour.

(c) Deafness

Sensorineural deafness almost always has a high frequency element and therefore frequently presents as a high frequency loss, eg. failure to hear the telephone bell. A high frequency loss commonly causes loss of speech discrimination ability.

(d) Tinnitus

"Tinnitus" refers to any sound heard in the ear itself. The external and middle ear sounds are crackling, popping or gurgling in character and may often be induced by manipulation of the ear or by auto–inflating the eustachian tube. The inner ear produces characteristic electronic–type sounds: humming, buzzing or ringing.

(e) Vertigo

Rotatory vertigo is the classic dizziness associated with ear disease. Blackouts or syncope are rarely due to ear disease and if these are present, closer enquiries regarding central nervous system symptoms should be made.

2.2 PHYSICAL EXAMINATION

A clear external canal is essential for adequate ear examination. Given an adequate view of the eardrum and a thorough history, most external and middle ear diseases can be diagnosed readily.

INSPECTION (handle the patient gently).

(a) Pinna

(include a postaural check for surgical scars)

(b) External meatus

(i) Straighten the canal by pulling the pinna posterolaterally – this reduces the overhang of the conchal bowl cartilage. The canal angles forward approximately 40 degrees and often also upwards. The drum is readily located by following the anterior wall of the canal.

(ii) Examine with an auriscope (ensure it has a bright light and fresh batteries).

(iii) Clean the external canal if required (See chapter on Cleaning the Ear).

(iv) Re–examine.

(c) Eardrum

The entire drum is not usually seen through one view of the auriscope and a composite view in the mind's eye is obtained by moving the field of vision around. A 4mm speculum is usually optimal. This size is the largest one able to fit into most external canals.

(i) Shape

The tympanic membrane should have a shallow curved loudspeaker shape. Local areas of atrophy and retraction are common after infection and grommet insertions. Chronic eustachian insufficiency results in retraction, then collapse of the drum. This collapse begins in the posterosuperior quadrant and extends to involve the entire tympanic membrane. In this condition, severe adhesive otitis, the drum takes on the consistency of "kitchen wrap" and becomes draped over the middle ear structures. Localised retractions of the pars flaccida area are relatively common. However, crusting and debris accumulation in association with such retractions are to be treated with suspicion as these may indicate the development of cholesteatoma (See Chapter VII). Granulations on the tympanic membrane are frequently associated with chronic middle ear disease, and should be approached with a high degree of suspicion.

(ii) Colour

The normal tympanic membrane is a pale grey, transparent shade with perhaps a pink or beige tint but with age, the drum becomes somewhat milky in appearance. Patches of chalky material in the tympanic membrane are due to tympanosclerosis. In the absence of deafness these are not clinically significant. Bubbles and fluid levels in retrotympanic fluid may be present but are usually difficult to see. Knowledge of the normal appearance is important. Subtle colour or transparency changes are frequent signs of the more common middle ear conditions.

(iii) Mobility, Autoinflation

A mobile tympanic membrane tested with a pneumatic speculum indicates little or no fluid in the middle ear. Using autoinflation as a test of eustachi-

an tubal patency (Valsalva manoeuvre) is not reliable as many normal people cannot perform this manoeuvre efficiently.

2.3 EXAMINATION OF HEARING

(a) Vocal Testing

A preliminary assessment of a patient's hearing can be gained by testing his ability to hear the examiner's voice at graded levels of loudness. The table below gives a rough guide to the patient's ability to hear the examiner's voice at about one metre, in quiet surroundings. The examiner's mouth should be hidden to prevent lipreading and the contralateral ear is masked with rustling paper.

Voice Loudness Level	Approximate Level of Hearing
Whisper	0–15db
Soft Voice	25–30db
Conversation	35–40db
Loud Voice	45–55db
Shout	60–70db

(b) Tuning Fork Tests

Two tests are performed: (i) Weber
(ii) Rinne

(i) The Weber test is performed by pressing the vibrating fork to the midline of the skull (forehead or vertex). In normal subjects the sound is described as being heard "in the middle" or "all over" (Weber "central"). The tone is heard in the better ear in sensorineural deafness and in the worse ear in conductive deafness.

(ii) The Rinne test is performed by holding the vibrating fork vertically three centimetres lateral to the external meatus, with the arms of the fork in a line directly lateral from the ear. The patient is instructed to listen to the sound, and the fork is then transferred immediately to the mastoid process and pressed firmly on the bone. The patient is then asked which is the louder sound. The first is louder (positive test) in normal ears or in sensorineural deafness. The second mastoid tone is louder (negative test) in conductive deafness although false negatives can occur in which the bone conduction is heard in the normal contralateral ear. (Figs. 8(a), (b), (c), (d), (e)).

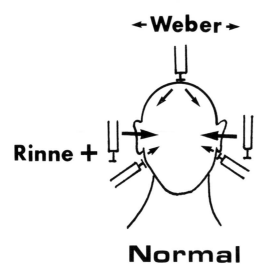

Normal

Figure 8(a). Normal tuning fork tests. The Weber is central and the Rinne is positive in both ears.

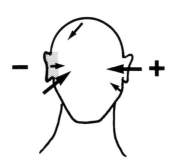

Conductive

Figure 8(b). Conductive deafness. The Weber refers to the deaf ear (shaded). The Rinne is positive in the normal ear, negative in the deaf ear.

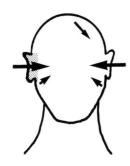

Sensorineural

Figure 8(c). Sensorineural deafness. The Weber refers to the better ear. The Rinne test is positive in both sides.

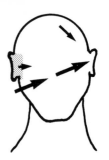

False-ve Rinne

Figure 8(d). False negative Rinne test. This is a phenomenon sometimes seen in cases of severe unilateral sensorineural deafness. The bone conduction element of the Rinne test is heard in the contralateral better ear. This superficially resembles a negative Rinne but the Weber refers to the better ear, not the deaf ear as in conductive deafness.

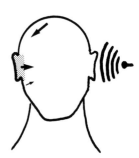

Masking Effect

Figure 8(e). Effect of masking on a false negative Rinne test. Masking the better ear abolishes the false negative effect.

2.4 AUDIOMETRY

Tests of Function: These are tests of the auditory and vestibular systems.

(a) Hearing

Measures of auditory function assist in the differentiation of conductive, cochlear and central hearing impairment. Tests include pure tone audiometry (PTA), basic measures of speech discrimination, middle ear measures, auditory evoked potentials (AEP), complex site of lesion tests, and measures of central auditory processing. These test procedures are being increasingly performed by audiologists who are scientists with specialist training in complex hearing assessment and rehabilitation.

(i) Pure Tone Audiometry (PTA)

The PTA is the most basic measure of hearing and shows acuity by providing a graph of the loudness threshold or hearing level in decibels (db) versus frequency (250 Hertz to 8,000 Hertz). This graph or audiogram shows the individual ear air conduction threshold, which is obtained using specially calibrated headphones, and the bone conduction threshold, obtained by directly stimulating the cochlea using a vibrator placed on the mastoid. In conductive deafness, the bone conduction thresholds are normal, but air conduction thresholds deteriorate, producing an air–bone gap. In sensorineural deafness, impairments of cochlear function cause a deterioration in both air and bone thresholds. Mixed deafness is a combination of the two. Note that conductive deafness always has a low frequency component, whereas sensorineural deafness almost always has a high frequency component.

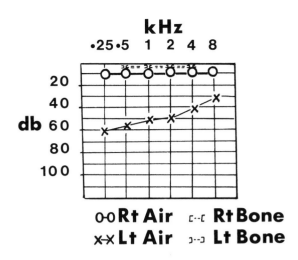

Figure 9(c). Conductive deafness. Left ear. The air conduction levels have sunk considerably to sixty decibels but the bone conductions remain normal. The "air/bone gap" between the bone conduction and air conduction levels represents the conductive loss which may be repaired.

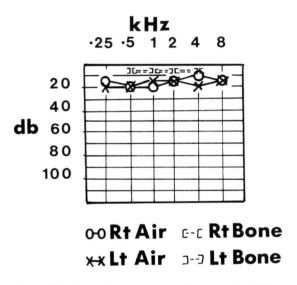

Figure 9(a). Normal pure tone audiometry. In children hearing levels are between five to ten decibels, later in life these levels may sink to approximately fifteen to twenty decibels.

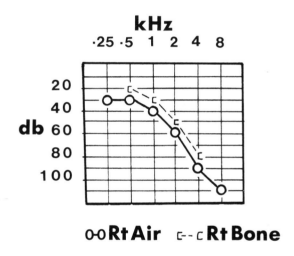

Figure 9(d). Sensorineural deafness. Both the bone conduction and air conduction levels have fallen in the high frequencies. This is a pattern common to many inner ear diseases.

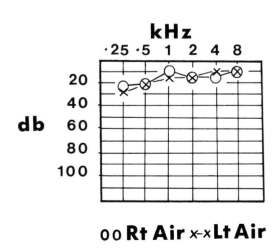

Figure 9(b). Minor low frequency losses commonly found in imperfect testing situations.

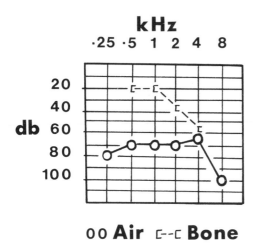

kHz

oo **Air** ⸦--⸧ **Bone**

Figure 9(e). Mixed deafness. A conductive deafness is present with an air/bone gap of fifty decibels in the low frequencies. In the high frequencies the bone conduction levels have fallen indicative of a sensorineural loss. The pattern is typical of many cases of chronic otitis media.

    (ii) Auditory Evoked Potentials (AEP)

Electrical activity is recorded from the auditory pathway in response to "click" or tone burst stimuli using computer averaging. The two main procedures are ECoG (Electrocochleography), which is recorded from the cochlea, usually transtympanically, and ABR (Auditory Brainstem Response), audiometry which records the potentials in the first 10 milliseconds post–stimulus. Both procedures provide an objective indication of hearing levels but are more commonly applied diagnostically: ECoG provides information on cochlear fluid pressures, and ABR provides a wave pattern related to conduction in the auditory nerve and brain stem. Hence ABR is the method choice in differentiating between sensory (ie. cochlear) and neural (ie. VIII nerve) deafness.

(b) Eustachian Tube Function: Tympanometry/Immittance

This assesses the elasticity (or "compliance") of the tympanic membrane by means of a low frequency sonar probe. When sound from the probe strikes the tympanic membrane, part of the sound is absorbed and part is reflected. (Figs. 10(a)(b))

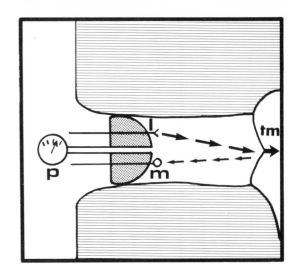

Figure 10(a). Principals of tympanometry. Sound is directed at the tympanic membrane from the loudspeaker (l). Part is absorbed by the middle ear mechanism and part is reflected back to the probe where it is detected by the microphone (m). The pressure in the external canal can be varied by the pressure pump (p).

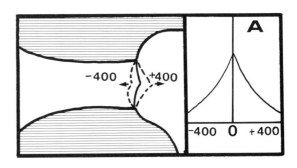

Figure 10(b). Type A tympanometry curve. Normal middle ear pressure. The compliance curve peaks when the external canal pressure equals the middle ear pressure at atmospheric pressure.

Absorption is maximal when the tympanic membrane is least taut, i.e. when the pressure in the middle ear equals that outside. If pressure changes inside the ear place the tympanic membrane under tension, more sound is reflected. The tympanometer probe is therefore equipped with an emitting loud speaker and a recording microphone. In addition, an air–tight seal and pump provide variable pressure in the external meatus, (from $+400$mm H_2O to -400mm H_2O) which is continually monitored. By measuring compliance against pressure, the middle ear pressure can be assessed as the compliance will be maximal when the known external meatus pressure equals the middle ear pressure. Normal or negative intra–tympanic pressure can therefore be ascertained. When the middle ear is filled with fluid, as in "glue ear", the compliance remains unchanged, as the tympanic membrane is "splinted" by the incompressible fluid. (Figs. 10(c)(d), 11)

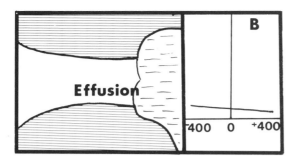

Figure 10(c). Type B tympanometry curve. Middle ear effusion. The compliance of the tympanic membrane varies little due to the inflexible nature of the middle ear fluid.

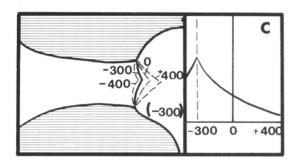

Figure 10(d). Type C tympanometry curve. Tubal insufficiency with a middle ear pressure of minus three hundred millimetres. Compliance is maximal when the external canal pressure equals the negative middle ear pressure.

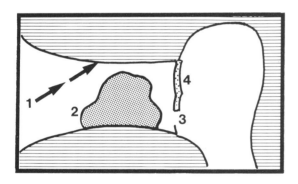

Figure 11. Aetiology of false Type B tympanometry curves.
1. Sound–beam misdirected.
2. Wax or debris in the external canal.
3. Perforated tympanic membrane.
4. Sclerosed tympanic membrane.

Reflex testing: If the tympanometry probe sound volume is raised, the tensor tympani and stapedius muscle contract when the sound perceived by the cochlea reaches 70 decibels. Contraction of these muscles alters the tympanic membrane compliance and therefore allows reading of the sound levels at which the reflexes come into play, together with their duration of action. This phenomenon is valuable in testing children's hearing for undetected losses and in acoustic neuroma when the reflexes decay or fade faster than normal.

(c) **Vestibular testing**
The function of the vestibular balance mechanisms is assessed by electronystagmography (ENG). Abnormal or uneven vestibular activity produces rhythmic flicking of the eyes – nystagmus. The cornea of the eye is positively charged relevant to the retina and the movement of the eye can therefore be measured by electrodes placed medially and laterally to the eye. The ENG provides a permanent record, similar to an electrocardiogram. Several effects are studied:

(i) Gaze direction
Change of direction of nystagmus with change of direction of the patient's eyes is suggestive of a central nervous system lesion.

(ii) Neck Positions
Nystagmus can be induced by changes in neck position causing vascular ischaemia due to vertebral artery compression. Nystagmus on such changes of position is recorded on the tracings.

(iii) Caloric testing

Under standard conditions the lateral semi–circular canals are stimulated with water at 44°C and 30°C respectively. A labyrinthine paresis results in reduced responses in the labyrinth tested.

(iv) Optic fixation
Nystagmus due to labyrinthine causes may be reduced or abolished by the eye fixing on a given point. This effect is readily recorded on the ENG.

2.5 OTHER INVESTIGATIONS

(a) **Radiology**
Radiological assessments may be required to assess ear disease itself or other causative conditions (eg. sinusitis). Plain films, CT scans, MRI scans and contrast studies (CNS or vascular) may all be required.

(b) **Microbiology**
Ear swabs, tests for syphilis, HIV.

(c) **Haematology**
Sensorineural deafness can occur in a variety of general illnesses, particularly autoimmune diseases, myxoedema and viral infections. The appropriate haematological tests may be indicated to detect these conditions.

CHAPTER 2:
OTALGIA

1. INTRODUCTION

Earache is a common cause of presentation, but many cases are not due to the ear itself. Adequate examination of the ear and a knowledge of other conditions which may mimic true otalgia will simplify the diagnosis in most cases.

2. HISTORY

The nature of otalgia is established by history taking as used with pain anywhere in the body. As previously discussed, interrogation should examine:

(a) The site of the otalgia as perceived by the patient is important. Many subjects will discern between a deep pain in the ear itself and a pain felt more on moving or touching the pinna (as in otitis externa) or in moving the jaw (e.g. in temporomandibular joint arthralgia.)

(b) The onset of pain should be linked if possible to any known causative factors. For instance, a recent upper respiratory tract infection may indicate a middle ear site. Swimming in summer often causes otitis externa. A prior tonsillectomy frequently results in referred otalgia.

(c) Otalgia of long duration tends to indicate a chronic condition, eg. malignancy, as opposed to the short history of, for example, acute otitis media.

(d) The nature of the pain helps suggest the site of origin. A dull ache may suggest inflammatory processes in immobile tissues, as opposed to sharp acute pain resulting from movement of sensitive tissues. The latter occurs in auto–inflation during acute otitis media, which induces more tension upon an already stretched and sensitive tympanic membrane.

(e) The severity of the pain may help to indicate the degree to which a condition has progressed. Severe furunculosis of the external meatus may produce exquisite pain, particularly during traction on the pinna. This is due to the canal skin being stretched tightly by oedema and pus under pressure.

(f) The frequency of episodes in cases of intermittent pain may suggest improvement or worsening of the condition and may therefore influence the treatment decided upon (e.g. in a child suffering repeated bouts of increasing frequency due to eustachian insufficiency, early surgical intervention by grommet insertion may be indicated to abort further episodes).

(g) The presence of aggravating or relieving factors may help significantly in localising the source of pain. Movement of the pinna greatly increases the pain of acute otitis externa and perichondritis, whereas jaw movement may cause an exacerbation of temporomandibular joint arthralgia.

(h) Associated symptoms. The presence or absence of the other cardinal symptoms of ear disease (discharge, deafness, tinnitus, vertigo) is ascertained, as their presence may indicate true otologic otalgia. Care must be taken to ensure that the patient is not confused with apparent rather than real deafness in such conditions as TM joint arthralgia, which may give rise to a sensation of blockage in the ear as opposed to true deafness. Symptoms due to other disease, such as upper respiratory tract infection, may indicate a cause for the otalgia.

(i) Radiation of the pain to the ear is a common cause of otalgia due to distant sites. Such radiation is common in dental disease, during the post–tonsillectomy period and in many pharyngeal malignancies or abscesses.

3. EXAMINATION

Given a good view of the tympanic membrane, it is reasonable to say that the cause of all true otological earache can be seen by careful inspection of the external ear and tympanic membrane. Difficulty may arise in badly scarred or tympanosclerotic tympanic membranes, but the great majority of painful ear conditions exhibit characteristic features. If the ear appears normal, suspect a non–otological cause and carefully examine the periotic or distant sites of referred otalgia.

(a) External Ear

Inspection and manipulation of the pinna reveals or excludes tenderness related to its movement. Painful canal conditions such as furunculosis or otomycosis are easily seen if the ear canal is free of wax debris.

(b) Tympanic Membrane

Tympanic membrane inspection and the appearance of the clinical conditions causing earache (eustachian insufficiency, viral myringitis, middle ear infections) are covered in the chapters on these conditions. Note that a clear, unimpeded view of the tympanic membrane is essential. If the tympanic membrane and canal are clear of overt causes of otalgia, inspect the periotic areas. Of these, the temporomandibular joint is the most common culprit. The joint is examined carefully (as below), then the parotid and local lymph nodes are assessed.

(c) Other Sites

A thorough examination of the nose and postnasal space, mouth, pharynx, larynx, neck and cervical spine is undertaken to exclude sites supplied by V2, IX, X, XI, C1, C2, C3, to exclude sites of origin of referred pain.

4. CONDITIONS COMMONLY CAUSING OTALGIA

4.1 EAR

(a) External: Perichondritis

Bacterial otitis externa

Furunculosis

Otomycosis

Viral myringitis

Trauma

(b) Middle Ear: Acute eustachian insufficiency

Acute otitis media

Chronic otitis media and cholesteatoma

Acute mastoiditis

(c) Others: Carcinoma of the ear

Herpes zoster oticus

Petrositis

4.2 PERIOTIC CAUSES (Fig. 12a)

(a) Temporomandibular joint arthralgia

(b) Parotitis

(c) Node inflammation

(d) Temporal arteritis

4.3 DISTAL SITES

(a) V2, V3 Sinusitis
Dental abscesses
Carcinoma of the mouth

(b) IX Carcinoma of the tonsil (Fig. 13)
Post–tonsillectomy
Quinsy

(c) X Carcinoma of the hypopharynx and larynx (Fig. 14)
Acute infections
Trauma

(d) C1, C2, C3 Cervical spine
Deep cervical structure inflammation or damage

5. PERIOTIC CONDITIONS

5.1 TEMPOROMANDIBULAR JOINT ARTHRALGIA

Pain from the temporomandibular joint can arise from either acute or chronic causes. Acute arthralgia, often in low grade recurrent form, is a common result of stress effects on the head and neck (along with tension headaches and globus syndromes). The aetiology is often bruxism, or clenching and grinding of teeth whilst asleep. The patient often gives a history of being under stress and may have noted a tendency to grit his teeth. Dental malocclusion may initiate or exacerbate the condition as a result of abnormal stress on the joints during dental occlusion and mastication. Chronic temporomandibular joint pain may arise from the prolonged acute state or from the general arthritis group (osteoarthritis, rheumatoid arthritis, trauma.)

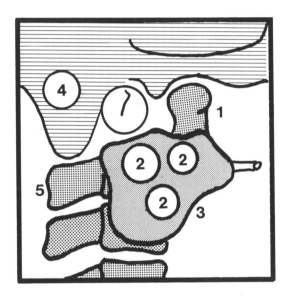

Figure 12(a). Aetiology of periotic otalgia.
1. Temporomandibular joint dysfunction.
2. Periotic nodes.
3. Acute parotitis.
4. Postauricular lymphadenitis.
5. Local musculoskeletal inflammation.

(a) *Examination*

Examination shows pain over the joint or its musculature, the latter being due to muscle spasm. Tenderness in the joint is palpated laterally over the disc, and posteriorly over the anterior external meatal wall. The latter is achieved by insertion of the little finger into the external meatus. The tenderness is maximal during joint movement. Tenderness over the temporalis and its insertion, the masseter and the pterygoids (submandibular and buccal cavity palpation) may signify further evidence of muscular spasm.

(b) *Management*

Management of TMJ arthralgia is to eliminate the immediate symptoms followed by correction of the causative factors. Pain is relieved by analgesia and anti–arthritics, eg. piroxicam 20mg nocte; sulindac 200mg b.d. and by elimination of muscular spasm by means of nocte diazepam 5mg. To avoid misunderstanding the patient should be warned that the use of the diazepam is to obtain muscle relaxation rather than the normal tranquilliser effect, the latter being interpreted by the layman as being for "nerves". The management of dental malocclusion is best undertaken by a specialist prosthodontist or oral surgeon and remains a controversial field. Filing of contact points and fitting of occlusal splints are employed to correct dental pathology. Arthritis due to other causes (osteoarthritis, rheumatoid arthritis) is managed as usual for these conditions.

5.2 PAROTITIS

Presents as an enlarged parotid with or without tenderness. Minor enlargements can often be best assessed by palpation of the parotid tail situated inferiorly to the pinna. Radiology, including sialography, will help establish the diagnosis.

6. REFERRED OTALGIA

Due to the complex innervations of the ear, referred otalgia can arise from most sites in the head and neck. The references above illustrate most instances and comment will be made on only a few. Post–tonsillectomy otalgia is the rule rather than the exception to such a degree that previous authors have commented on the need to check the ears to avoid missing a cause of true otalgia. Temporomandibular joint pain due to the mouth gag used in tonsillectomy may contribute in this group. Deep dental pain is a frequent cause of otalgia not readily detected on many occasions. An orthopantomogram (OPG) may help in these cases. In the elderly, earache in the absence of readily detected ear or temporomandibular joint origin may suggest a more deep–rooted pathology, possibly throat malignancy, and should be regarded with suspicion. (Figs. 12(b), 13, 14)

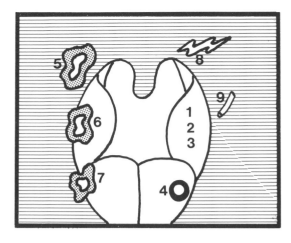

Figure 13. Pharyngeal causes of referred otalgia.(Glossopharyngeal)

1. Tonsillitis.
2. Quinsy.
3. Tonsillectomy.
4. Aphthous ulceration.
5. Palatal carcinoma.
6. Tonsillar carcinoma.
7. Lingual carcinoma.
8. Palatal trauma.
9. Glossopharyngeal neuralgia.

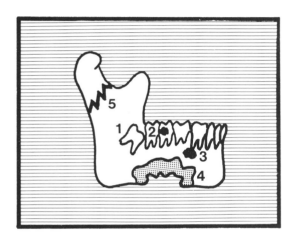

Figure 12(b). Mandibular causes of otalgia (V3)
1. Wisdom tooth pathology.
2. Dental caries.
3. Apical abscess.
4. Mandibular carcinoma.
5. Trauma.

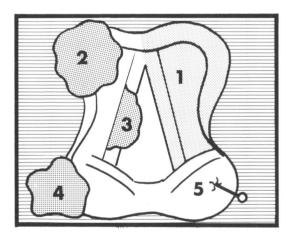

Figure 14. Hypopharyngeal causes for referred otalgia (vagal).

1. Acute epiglottitis.

2. Supraglottic carcinoma.

3. Laryngeal carcinoma.

4. Piriform fossa carcinoma.

5. Hypopharyngeal trauma.

CHAPTER 3:
CLEANING THE EAR

Removal of debris in the EAM to obtain a full view of the tympanic membrane frustrates many practitioners. It is a technique which can only be mastered with practice and is often poorly taught. The usual problems are lack of equipment, poor lighting, and the sensitivity of the deep canal. Nevertheless, even with only limited equipment and lighting, combined with a gentle touch and good patient rapport, success is the rule rather than exception.

1.   TECHNIQUES AVAILABLE

1.1 SYRINGING

1.2 SUCTION

1.3 INSTRUMENTAL REMOVAL

(a) Wool carrier

(b) Wax loops or hooks

(c) Microforceps

1.1 SYRINGING

In the primary care situations, syringing is the most common technique of ear cleaning. It must not be used if the presence of a drum perforation is possible for fear of contaminating the middle ear and mastoid cells with infected debris. A 200ml syringe or a continuous (Bacon) syringe is used. The patient is draped with a waterproof sheet and towel and a kidney dish is held under the ear to catch the flushings. Water at 37°C is used to avoid vertigo. The canal is examined to establish the site of the debris. Water is then flushed around one side of (not at) the debris until this is dislodged. Whilst syringing, the canal is straightened by pulling the pinna posterolaterally. The syringe is steadied by an extended small finger placed against the skull. It is important to mop the canal dry at the conclusion. (Fig. 15)

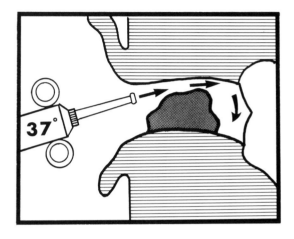

Figure 15.   Syringing technique. The stream of water should be directed around the occluding mass and should avoid direct pressure on the tympanic membrane. Note that the irrigating fluid should be maintained at 37°C.

Problems:

(a) Poor draping may result in a soaked patient.

(b) Hot or cold water may cause unpleasant vertigo.

(c) Failure to steady the syringe may result in trauma to the external meatus or drum.

(d) Obstinate hard wax or keratosis may resist prolonged syringing – instrumental removal will be required.

(e) Poor removal of debris may cause secondary otitis externa.

(f) Middle ear infection may result from irrigation due to a previously undetected drum perforation.

(g) A drum perforation may result from directly syringing the tympanic membrane, particularly if this has been previously weakened.

1.2 SUCTION TOILET

Cleaning of fluid or semi–fluid debris by suction is the technique preferred by most otologists. Suction is derived from an electric or gas pump, or from a water–operated pump attached to a tap. A range of suckers is available commercially, including some inexpensive lightweight plastic/metal designs. Good lighting is necessary because of the relatively sharp metal tips of the suckers. Optimally, the patient lies supine, his head steady on a pillow. The canal is straightened with a speculum and the sucker hand is steadied against the skull. The canal is cleaned laterally to medially with particular care in the region of the tympanic membrane. A peeling action is used to strip away dead skin and debris. Irrigation with lukewarm water or saline may help to soften or remove more solid debris.

Problems:

(a) Suction may be extremely noisy and this may disturb children.

(b) Good lighting is essential.

(c) Delicacy is required to avoid deep canal discomfort.

(d) Mild vertigo may occur after prolonged suction due to a cold air stream affecting the lateral semi–circular canal.

1.3 INSTRUMENTAL REMOVAL

(a) Dry mopping

(i) Wool Carriers

Soft wax or fluid debris may be cleaned with cotton wool twisted tightly onto a stiff carrier. The latter may be roughened stiff wire, a thin flattened (Jobson–Horne) probe, or lacking these, a thin wooden stick whittled down to about a 2mm diameter.

Technique: In each case a small amount of wool is twisted tightly around the carrier and doubled over the sharp ends to protect the patient from injury. The swab should be about 3mm diameter, 15mm long and with 2–3mm of wool overlap at the end. Before use, tap the end of the swab on a finger to check for the presence of an inadvertent sharp point. Multiple swabs may be required to clean the canal thoroughly. The cleaning hand is steadied with the little finger on the skull. Cleaning is begun at the surface, then progressively down the canal. Dried crusting at the entrance is softened and removed with wet swabbing. The swab is gently twirled in the hand, moving around the canal wall to gently scour debris off the canal skin. Particular care is taken near the sensitive tympanic membrane. The swab is rotated in the direction which will tighten the wool on the carrier, otherwise the wool will unwind and come off in the canal. (Fig. 16)

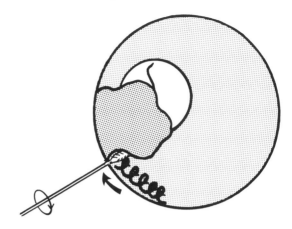

Figure 16. Use of the wool carrier to clear debris from the external auditory canal. The carrier is twirled in the fingers whilst moved around the external canal wall, elevating the debris away from the wall.

(ii) Hockey Stick

Debris in the anterior recess (the angle between the tympanic membrane and the anterior wall) may be difficult to approach. In this case, fashion a narrow tight swab and angle the last 2–3mm, which has no rigid metal core, to about 45^0. This is then inserted into the floor of the recess and rotated upwards, dislodging the debris. (Figs. 17(a)(b)).

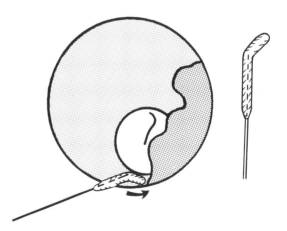

Figure 17(a). Use of the "hockey stick" wool carrier. The distal two millimetres of the tightly wound wool is angled to gain access to the anterior recess.

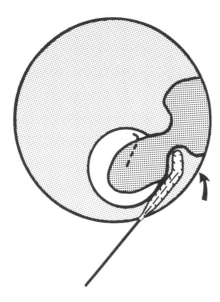

Figure 17(b). The "hockey stick" is gently rotated through the anterior recess lifting the debris out of the pocket.

(b) Wax Loops, Wax Hooks

Fine loops or hooks are commercially available for removing firm or hard wax.

(i) Loops

Loops are used to gently dislodge debris and to draw the dislodged material to the surface. They optimally incorporate a 5mm ellipse of fine high tensile wire approximately 2–3mm in diameter and angled $10-20^{\circ}$ on the shaft. They are used to gently dislodge debris and draw it to the surface. Use the loop to lift adherent skin or scale off the canal wall prior to removal. (Figs. 18(a)(b)).

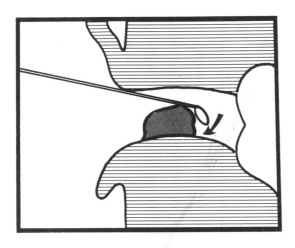

Figure 18(a). Use of the aural loop. The loop is angled and gently introduced past the debris in the external canal.

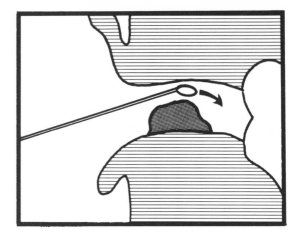

Figure 18(b). The debris is removed by elevating the handle of the loop and gently withdrawing the debris. Care should be observed to avoid trauma to the canal wall.

(ii) Hooks

Hooks are used to remove tough debris and foreign bodies. They are manoeuvred around the object and then rotated to site the tip behind the mass, which is then drawn out. Care must be observed not to gouge the canal on withdrawal. (Fig. 19).

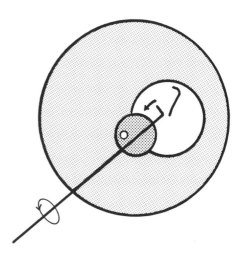

Figure 19.   Use of the aural hook to remove a foreign body in the deep canal. The hook is gently introduced past the foreign body, rotated and withdrawn.

(c) Forceps

Fine alligator or cupped forceps are of particular use in removal of fine scale or similar adherent debris. Because of the thin pointed ends, good visualisation is required, eg. via an auriscope or microscope.

2. LIGHTING

Lack of good vision is the usual frustration in cleaning the ear. Adequate lighting of the work area is essential. One of the methods below is usually available and all these techniques have a common objective: to provide a beam of light which is as coaxial as possible with the line of vision. Full mobility and the use of both hands is desirable.

2.1 FLASHLIGHT

In the absence of other means, a powerful light held close to the examiner's right ear by an assistant will suffice. In order to avoid angulation of the light beam the examiner will need to work about 60cm from the patient.

2.2 AURISCOPE

These have an advantage of being readily available with a built–in speculum (use 4mm or larger if possible). The light is nearly coaxial. A good bulb and fresh batteries are mandatory. The magnifying glass is removed during the cleaning procedure. An auriscope has the disadvantage of being cumbersome to stabilise. It may provide limited access because of the design of certain brands, and use of the second hand is limited.

2.3 HEAD MIRROR

This, the most famous tool–of–trade of the Otolaryngologist, has the advantages of coaxial light, good surgeon mobility and free use of both hands. Its popularity within the specialty reflects these advantages. Mastery of the mirror is not difficult but requires patience. Note that the light is placed 30cm to the right of and above the patient, with the beam played fully on the surgeon's face. The mirror, when sited correctly, allows vision by the right eye through the centre of the mirror whilst shielding both eyes from the light. The disadvantage of the mirror is a limited range of head movement by the surgeon, requiring mirror or light adjustments if positional changes are required, although this is not usual in ear cleaning (Fig. 20). If a patient is mobile (eg. a child), rest the patient on a pillow or against the mother's chest.

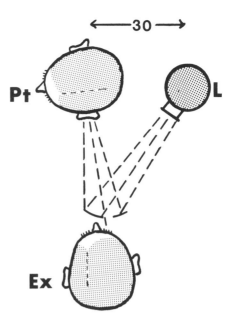

Figure 20.   Use of the head mirror. Note that the light should be thirty centimetres to the right of and above the subject. This permits good coaxial vision without the examiner being blinded by the light.

2.4 HEADLIGHT

These are more easily mastered than the mirror, although the light beam may not be quite so coaxial. Greater range of movement during examination is also possible. The disadvantages are that the light is heavier and requires attachment to a power source. This must be disconnected after each examination, or, if carried on the body, is often cumbersome, as the light lead tends to become entangled. Fibreoptic lights are even more cumbersome.

2.5 OPERATING MICROSCOPE

Originally introduced specifically for otology, the microscope is the great advantage of the specialist over the primary care physician. Superb coaxial light is combined with a choice of magnifications, excellent optics and mobility, and full use of both hands. Together with microsuction techniques, it allows state–of–the–art cleaning and diagnosis. The disadvantage is the cost.

3. USE OF THE EAR WICK

An ear wick – a length of cotton gauze inserted into the external canal – is a common technique used in the management of otitis externa and some middle ear conditions. A wick is used for several purposes:

(a) **Oedema** – Firm pressure from a wick abolishes canal oedema, particularly in the superficial areas, thus permitting visualisation and cleaning of the deep canal.

(b) The wick may be used as a **vector** to carry antimicrobial preparations deep into the canal.

(c) The cotton has a gentle **hygroscopic action** to absorb excess moisture in the canal.

(d) A wick may be used to **maintain a deposit** of preparation (eg. antibiotic cream) in the canal, particularly in patients who may be unreliable in carrying out repeated topical medication applications.

3.1 METHOD OF INSERTION

(a) Wick Size

Unless the patient has a large canal, the standard (10–12mm) gauze strip is too wide for thorough insertion. Accordingly, divide the gauze strip longitudinally to form a long narrow strip. This is particularly necessary in cases of canal oedema. Approximately 20–30cm is adequate.

(b) Site preparation

The canal is cleaned as adequately as conditions permit, by suction or dry mopping. If a cream or ointment is to be used, this is gently worked into the deep canal with a narrow twist of cotton wool on a carrier, or is impregnated into the wick itself. The author prefers the former technique as being simpler.

(c) Insertion Technique

The direction of the external canal is ascertained by inspection. The wick is grasped in fine forceps longitudinally 5–10mm from the end and is gently introduced, waving the forcep tips slightly to judge the canal direction by touch. The wick is inserted about 3cm, i.e. to within about 5–10mm from the membrane. (Fig. 21(a)) The wick is then gently released, the forceps are withdrawn 1cm, and the wick is then re–grasped and advanced a further centimetre. A back and forth packing action is continued (Fig. 21(b)), the wick being packed gradually firmer against the deeper packing. The canal fills and in the lateral (cartilaginous) part of the canal firm, but not hard, packing is used to reduce oedema. (Fig. 21(c)) The packing hand is rested on the skull throughout using the small finger. Generally antibiotic wicks are replaced in 2–3 days but wicks impregnated with more powerful agents (eg. gentamicin), may be left in for up to one week.

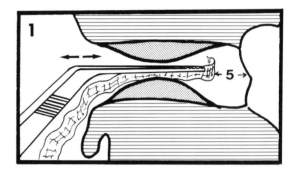

Figure 21(a). Use of the ear wick. A narrow ribbon gauze wick is gently introduced to within five millimetres of the tympanic membrane. The forceps are withdrawn several millimetres.

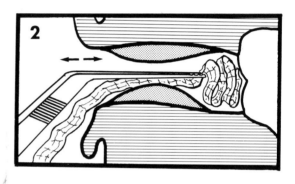

Figure 21(b). The gauze is regrasped and the deep canal is progressively packed by a gentle to and fro grasping and releasing action.

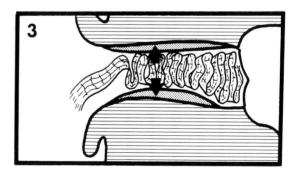

Figure 21(c). When fully packed the gauze exerts gentle pressure on the oedematous canal, eliminating the swelling and absorbing any effusion.

3.2 COMMOM PROBLEMS DURING WICK USE

(a) *Excessive thickness:*

A wide wick tends to "jam" in narrow canals, preventing insertion into the deep meatus. Longitudinal division creates a narrow wick which is more suitable in most cases.

(b) *Failure to insert a wick deeply:*

An initial inadequate insertion hinders further packing, resulting in only the superficial canal being packed. Hesitancy by the practitioner if working blind is understandable. However, if fine forceps are used, the tips are guarded as in Fig. 21(a), and the insertion is done gently, then damage is unlikely.

(c) *Canal wall trauma:*

This should be avoided by delicate technique, feeling one's way carefully and by bracing the packing hand against the head with the small finger.

(d) *Forceps pressure:*

When releasing the grip on the wick, avoid abrupt opening of the forceps as these will spring against the canal wall, causing extreme discomfort.

(e) *Wick expulsion or removal:*

Movement of the jaw and the temporomandibular joint may cause extrusion of part of the wick, particularly as the oedema resolves. Warn the patient of this possibility and advise him to cut off the extruding part or to retain it with a cotton wool plug. If a patient, particularly a child, is suspected of pulling the wick out, tape a cotton wool plug into the conchal bowl.

3.3 NON–RIBBON/TAMPON TYPE WICKS

Other techniques may be used to achieve some or all of the wick functions described above. The Merocel "Otowick" was developed as a slender tampon to absorb external auditory canal debris. Although easily inserted, these wicks are rigid and may cause trauma. Once saturated, the expanded wick material provides little pressure to reduce oedema. Porous hydrophilic polyurethane sponge may also be used. This is cut from sheets of "Allevyn" (Smith & Nephew), a commonly available burns dressings. Sections of 5x5x20mm are used. These wicks will swell to approximately double size when fully hydrated. The polyurethane is soft to touch and comfortable when inserted.

Technique: Clean the ear thoroughly, then instil the appropriate topical medication into the canal with a wool carrier. Use ointments rather than creams (the latter are absorbed rapidly into the wick and therefore reduce its hydroscopic action). Insert the wick with fine forceps. Removal is simple and can be performed by the patient's family or friends if necessary. If the canal is severely oedematous, use a thinner section than the above dimensions and replace after 24 hours. If a child is likely to attempt removal, cut the wick shorter and insert deeper to prevent self–removal.

Chapter 4:
Inherited Conditions

1. EMBRYOLOGY

All three compartments of the ear have complex origins. The ear structures take contributions from the ectoderm, mesoderm and endodermal sources.

(a) External

The pinna appears as small hillocks derived from the maxillo–mandibular (first) and hyoid (second) arches. These fuse to form a recognisable shape by the end of the second month.

The external meatus is derived from the first pharyngeal ectodermal groove and develops medially as a core of ectodermal cells which hollows out to form the canal.

(b) Eustachian Tube

The eustachian tube develops from the dorsal part of the first pharyngeal endodermal groove as the tubo–tympanic recess. The endoderm of the recess therefore comes to line the middle ear and mastoid cells.

The tympanic membrane derives its three layers from the ectoderm of the canal, mesoderm (its fibrous middle layer) and the endoderm of the tubo–tympanic recess.

The ossicles are derived from the first arch (Meckels) cartilage which provides the malleus and most of the incus, and the second arch (Reichert's) cartilage, which supplies the stapes and the tip of the incus long process. The ossicles are later enveloped in endoderm from the tubo–tympanic recess.

(c) Inner Ear

The membranous labyrinth develops as an ectodermal thickening (the otic placode) near the pinna. This sinks into the mesoderm forming the otic vesicle which then forms cochlear and vestibular pouches which go on to form the membranous labyrinth. The otic capsule forms from chondrification then ossification of the surrounding mesoderm.

The auditory nerve is derived from the acoustico–facial portion of the neural crest and is related to the otic vesicle from an early stage. (Fig 22)

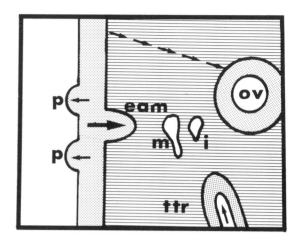

Figure 22. Embryology of the ear. The external canal arises from an epithelial ingrowth between the embryological pinna formation. The middle ear structures are mesodermal in origin and become enveloped in fine epithelium which develops from the tubo–tympanic recess (ttr). The inner ear is derived from the ectoderm which forms the otic vesicle which then sinks into the mesoderm. p: pinna; eam: external auditory meatus; m: malleus; i: incus; ov: otic vesicle.

2. ABERRANT STATES

Because of its complicated origin, aberrations of development are not infrequent. Major abnormalities are often associated with branchial arch syndromes:

Treacher–Collins
Pierre Robin
Crouzon's
Apert's
Goldenhars

3. EAR CONDITIONS

3.1 MINOR DEFORMITIES

(a) *Preauricular fistula*

(b) *Preauricular rudiments*

3.2 MAJOR DEFORMITIES

(a) *Microtia*

(b) *External canal atresia*

(c) *Middle ear agenesis*

(i) Tympanic membrane and ossicular malformations

(ii) Failure of aeration

(iii) Facial nerve aberrations

(d) *Inner ear deformities*

3.3 PROTRUDING (BAT) EARS

3.1 MINOR DEFORMITIES

(a) *Preauricular Fistula*

These are tracts of squamous epithelium, usually short sacs but sometimes widely ramifying into the parotid. These short sacs usually originate in the superior crus of the helix. Larger tracts may degenerate into a chronic fistula state, requiring excision. Removal requires a meticulous dissection technique, needed to avoid recurrence. The tract may be injected with Bonney's blue to aid this dissection.

(b) *Preauricular Rudiments*

Small pedunculated or sessile skin tags, some containing cartilage, may be found just anterior to the tragus. Ligate the base or excise as required.

3.2 MAJOR DEFORMITIES

Gross ear deformities frequently involve multiple compartments of the ear and are therefore considered together. Severe external malformations have a tendency to indicate inner ear aberrations also.

(a) *Microtia*

Failure of pinna development varies from mild shape abnormalities to mere skin tags at or near the meatal site. Gross pinna lesions are almost always associated with canal atresia and middle ear abnormalities.

(b) *Canal Atresia*

The canal site is marked by a shallow pit with soft tissue or a bony plate in the site of the meatus. The temporomandibular joint may sublux into the site of the canal, complicating reconstructive surgery.

(c) *Middle Ear Agenesis*

In cases of canal atresia, the tympanic membrane is usually obliterated with only a strand of the annulus present to suggest its site. Minor ossicular malformations in the absence of other congenital ear aberrations are an occasional finding and these may mimic otosclerosis. In cases of gross deformity the malleus and incus are often found to be fused and misshapen or perhaps fixed to the walls of the middle ear cleft. The stapes may be deformed, fixed or absent. Poor development of the eustachian tube may be present. This prevents middle ear aeration, and will frustrate tympanoplasty attempts. The middle ear cleft in these cases is found to be either not developed or filled with fibrous tissue. The facial nerve may be aberrant in its site and branches. This possibility renders exploration of congenital ears a painstaking and dangerous procedure.

(d) *Inner Ear*

A spectrum of abnormalities may be present, varying from mild membranous labyrinth deformities to gross otic capsule deformity or agenesis. Accompanying sensorineural losses vary from mild high frequency losses to total absence of hearing.

3.2.1 INVESTIGATIONS

(a) *Radiology*

Polytomography and high resolution CT scans help the surgeon to assess several features:

(i) The Nature of Canal Atresia
   The presence of a thick bony plate in the site of the canal will mean a longer procedure with painstaking drilling of a new canal. If the plate is thick, however, the temporomandibular joint is unlikely to sublux into the site of the canal.

(ii) Aeration of the Middle Ear
   Failure of aeration of the middle ear indicates a guarded prognosis with regards the possibility of hearing restoration from tympanoplasty efforts.

(iii) Ossicular state
   If well–shaped ossicles are present in a well–aerated middle ear, a better ossiculoplasty prognosis may be expected. Poorly shaped or absent ossicles will complicate surgical restoration of hearing.

(iv) Otic Capsule Malformations, particularly if severe, may indicate poor or absent cochlear function.

(v) Facial Nerve Aberrations may be detected by lateral tomograms and CT studies.

(b) Audiology

Speech development depends on hearing which must be assessed early in these cases. Computer–assisted audiometry (ABR, ECoG) and tympanometry (reflex testing) are used to assess the normal and abnormal ears. In unilateral cases, it is essential to establish that the apparently normal ear is functioning adequately as this will permit full intellectual development.

3.2.2 MANAGEMENT

(a) Cosmesis

Pinnaplasty, utilising local soft tissue, cartilage or synthetic implants, may be performed to produce an ear–like contour but the surgery is complex and may return results which are unsatisfactory to the patient. A prosthesis may be preferred, possibly with a longer hairstyle. Prostheses may be fastened with bone anchored mounts using transcutaneous titanium screws set into the skull itself. The aesthetic results of these prostheses are now frequently excellent.

(b) Hearing

Restoration of function via a meatoplasty and tympanoplasty (in gross cases) is a major challenge, and the results depend on the extent of the deformity. Creation of an external meatus with local skin grafts is of major benefit in bilateral cases. This allows the fitting of an air conduction aid capable of higher fidelity sound reproduction than is possible with bone conduction models. Bone anchored hearing aids may be combined with the cosmetic prostheses described above using the same titanium mounts. Results from these aids are very good if the cochlear function is normal. Because of the need for speech, surgery for hearing is undertaken early in bilateral cases, but is not essential in unilateral cases. In those cases in which deafness is a persisting or insuperable problem, full ancillary training to overcome the handicap of deafness is commenced. (See "Inner Ear Conditions: The Deaf Child").

3.3 PROTRUDING EARS

"Bat Ears" are due to one or more of several pinna cartilage variations.

(a) Excessive Conchal Bowl Depth

This causes the ear to stand away from the skull, causing a prominent but otherwise well–shaped ear.

(b) Antihelix Aberrations

Two problems may present: (Fig. 23)

(i) Superior crus – Failure of this fold development causes the upper pinna to fall laterally, causing the "elephant ear".

(ii) Kinking of the lower antihelix allows the ear to fold forwards, forming the "lop ear".

(c) Excessive Size of the Pinna Cartilage

Posterosuperior to the antihelix; results in a wing–like ear.

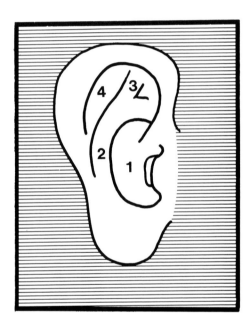

Figure 23.   Aetiology of protruding ears.
1. Excessive conchal cartilage bowl depth.
2. Failure of the antihelical contour.
3. Failure of the superior crus of the antihelix.
4. Excessive posterosuperior pinna cartilage formation.

3.3.1 PRESENTATION

Boys often present at 4–5 years of age when they are subjected to peer ridicule at school. Girls, after covering the ears with a longer hairstyle, may present later, at adolescence.

3.3.2 MANAGEMENT

One or more of the above abnormalities may be present. Surgery is tailored to the individual and incorporates the surgical procedures appropriate for the problem at hand.

(a) *The Conchal Bowl*

The medial bowl cartilage and soft tissues deep to the pinna are removed to allow the ear to move closer to the skull. (Fig. 24.1)

(b) *Antihelix*

By a posterior approach the aberrant areas are weakened then fixed with non–absorbent mattress sutures to restore contour. (Fig. 24.2)

(c) *Excessive Pinna Size*

This is more difficult to correct and a variety of more complex skin and cartilage reduction techniques is used.

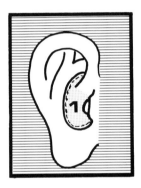 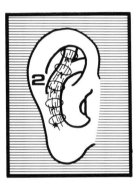

Figure 24.   Correction of protruding ears.
1. Excision of the deep conchal bowl cartilage.
2. Recreation of the antihelical contour.

CHAPTER 5:
CONDITIONS OF THE PINNA AND EXTERNAL AUDITORY MEATUS

1. PINNA

1.1 TRAUMA

The pinna is frequently subject to laceration or contusion injuries. Haematoma auris is a clot occurring between the pinna cartilage and its overlying perichondrium. It results from crushing or rolling injuries of the pinna and is prevalent amongst footballers and boxers. (See Chapter 9: Traumatic Conditions of the Ear)

1.2 INFECTIONS

Bacterial perichondritis of the auricle is usually due to staphylococcal or pseudomonal infections. It presents as an inflamed, exquisitely tender swelling. The condition is frequently a result of prior trauma, often minor, (eg. insect bite) or a result of otitis externa. If untreated, severe cartilage necrosis and deformity may result. Take a swab for culture and pending the results, begin the patient on high dose treatment to cover both likely pathogens. Combinations of flucloxacillin, cefaclor, ciprofloxacin and gentamicin are used initially, then the regime appropriate to the culture sensitivity results is continued. If fluctuation is present, surgical removal of the pus and necrotic cartilage is necessary, followed by careful tissue positioning and packing to maintain the cosmetic appearance of the ear.

1.3 NEOPLASMS

Squamous or basal cell carcinomas are prevalent amongst fair–skinned Europeans who have lived in the tropics. Lesions on the helical rim may be managed by excision of a through–and–through wedge including a margin of normal tissue, followed by direct closure. Larger lesions involving the central pinna require more radical excision. (Fig. 25)

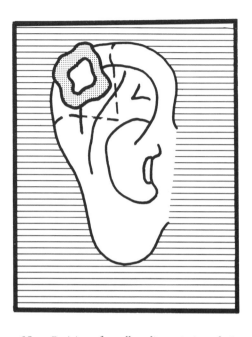

Figure 25.   Excision of small malignant pinna lesions. A through–and–through V–excision is undertaken allowing an adequate margin around the lesion. Approximation and closure will achieve an acceptable cosmetic result. Larger lesions will require more complex techniques.

2. EXTERNAL AUDITORY MEATUS

2.1 OTITIS EXTERNA

2.2 KERATOSIS OBTURANS

2.3 EXTERNAL CANAL TUMOURS

2.1 OTITIS EXTERNA

As a prelude to discussing this group of conditions, it should be noted that a common failure of management is the use of inappropriate topical preparations. Otitis externa, as with many skin conditions, involves aberrations of the moisture content of the skin. Treatments are therefore tailored to correct the situation at hand. All external ear infections should be managed with preliminary thorough cleaning of the pinna and canal.

Nature of Condition	Appropriate Remedy
Wet, weeping	Powders, pastes (moisture absorbent)
Moist	Creams (mildly hygroscopic)
Dry, scaling	Ointment (oil–based to retain moisture)

CLASSIFICATION OF OTITIS EXTERNA

2.1.1 SEBORRHOEIC

2.1.2 ALLERGIC

2.1.3 SEPTIC

(a) Bacterial
(i) Generalised

(ii) Neurodermatitis

(iii) Localised (furunculosis)

(b) Otomycosis

(c) Chronic myringitis

(d) Viral
(i) Herpes Zoster Oticus

(ii) Bullous myringitis

2.1.1 SEBORRHOEIC OTITIS EXTERNA

This is a dry, greasy, scaling inflammation of uncertain cause. It is usually associated with a greasy scalp and dandruff. Pruritis, and secondary infection from resultant self-trauma , are common. Management requires both scalp and ear care. The scalp is regularly shampooed to reduce grease content and remove dandruff. The use of hair oils is avoided. The external canal is cleaned by dry mopping or suction to remove debris and bacteria. Inflammation and infection are reduced with a steroid and antibiotic wick. The ear is re-cleaned in two days. The condition should stabilise within a week. Resistant cases are often due to scratching or rubbing – this should be discouraged (See "Neurodermatitis").

2.1.2 ALLERGIC OTITIS EXTERNA

(a) Aetiology
Allergens applied on or near the ear rapidly sensitise the super-fine skin of the canal and auricle. They may include hairsprays or other hair preparations and costume jewellery with its nickel content. Iatrogenic causes include penicillin and chloramphenicol ear drops (both obsolete), neomycin applications (still in common use) and iodine. Neomycin allergy produces an angry, diffuse swelling and reddening on and around the ear, superficially resembling erysipelas. Iodine produces marked swelling, erythema and a profuse serous discharge. Pain is common in both these allergies.

(b) Presentation
Pruritis is common and the ear may be excoriated and tender. Swelling, inflammation and discomfort may be present. Otorrhoea is often copious. A history of recent topical medication or a change in hair care may be forthcoming.

(c) Management
(i) The allergen is removed by meticulous cleaning of the pinna and external canal. If hair preparations are suspected, these are discarded. If nickel allergy is suspected, costume jewellery is discarded. Jewellery made of the "noble" metals (gold, silver, platinum) does not usually cause problems.

(ii) Reduce the inflammation with liberal applications of steroid cream.

(iii) Secondary infection is managed with topical antibacterials incorporated in the steroid cream, plus systemic amoxycillin or cefaclor.

(iv) A wick is used to minimise external canal oedema if present or to absorb copious discharge.

2.1.3 SEPTIC OTITIS EXTERNA

(a) Bacterial Otitis Externa
(i) Generalised

Diffuse bacterial otitis externa is usually due to staphylococcus, pseudomonas, streptococcus or gram negative organisms. Predisposing factors include the use of crowded or poorly maintained swimming pools during hot weather. The infections may also be initiated by minor trauma such as scratching or rubbing the external ear.

Presentation

Pruritis and gurgling in the ears are followed by pain and blockage. On examination the vestibule and external canal are sodden, inflamed and oedematous. Pain is noted on moving or pressing the pinna.

Management

Thorough canal cleaning is mandatory. Suction toilet is preferred but may be unavailable and is frequently distressing to children. In these circumstances use dry mopping. Cleaning the ear eliminates the bacteria themselves, nutrients and the moist environment.

Infection is managed with topical antibacterials (neomycin, polymixin, gramicidin), plus systemic antibiotics (amoxycillin/clavulanic acid or cefaclor). Gentamicin and steroid cream is used in resistant cases or where the blue-green debris of pseudomonal infection is present.

Reduce canal oedema by using an ear wick (see Cleaning the Ear). Most otitis externa cases are greatly relieved by the above management within 24 to 48 hours. Reclean the ear at 48 hours then a week later if progress is satisfactory.

(ii) Neurodermatitis is a form of bacterial otitis externa in which habitual rubbing or scratching of the ear is the main aetiological agent. These patients present with a red and swollen conchal bowl with cracking and peeling of the bowl skin adjacent to the entrance of the external canal. Canal inspection may show a fine, moist white discharge. Before initiating treatment, warn the patient that unless self–trauma ceases, treatment will be ineffective. Treat as for bacterial otitis externa, plus promethazine 10mg at night to reduce pruritis. Sometimes ear pads must be worn to bed for short periods during the healing phase to reduce trauma whilst asleep.

(iii) Furunculosis

Staphylococcus aureus may cause small (0.5cm) boil–like eruptions in the superficial canal hair follicles. The pus in the lesions is under considerable pressure. The condition ranks with perichondritis in its ability to cause severe otalgia.

Presentation

The patient may present in severe pain which is exacerbated by pinna manipulation or pressure. Scanty purulent otorrhoea may be noted. Severe canal oedema may be present. The pustules are seen in the superficial canal and multiple minor "carpet spread" lesions may be present.

Management

The canal is gently cleaned of discharge and gentamicin and steroid ointment is then worked into the depth of the canal with a very narrow cotton wool swab. A narrow wick is then used to gently pack the canal to reduce oedema. The wick is replaced two days later. High dose, anti–staphylococcal antibiotic cover is provided. Flucloxacillin, 500mg qid for one day, then 250mg qid is given, or cephalosporins in high dose in penicillin sensitive patients. Administration of gentamicin as a single dose (80mg for an adult) may be used to promote recovery. Strong pain relief is provided (codeine phosphate 30–60mg q4h, Mersyndol Forte, 2 q.i.d). The patient is warned that the pain will take approximately twenty–four hours to subside. Recovery should be complete after several days but the patient should be warned of the possibility of recurrence.

(b) *Otomycosis*

Fungal otitis externa is due usually to Aspergillus nigra, Aspergillus flavum or Candida albicans. The presentation is similar to bacterial otitis externa, but in many cases there is a history of unsuccessful management. On inspection, the fungal mass is readily observed. Aspergillus nigra has a dirty brown or black appearance, possibly with visible black or chocolate–coloured spores or mycelia present. Aspergillus flavum exhibits a yellow or orange–coloured debris. Candida has a white, furry appearance with a "wet blotting paper" texture of the debris. Thorough cleaning of these lesions is essential. Optimally, suction toilet is used to remove the debris and to peel out the dead skin lining the canal which frequently harbours the fungus. Adequate cleaning of the anterior recess is often difficult and may require a "hockey stick" swab. (See "Cleaning the Ear"). Combinations of antifungal preparations are used to minimise the likelihood of recurrence. Nystatin, clotrimazole, econazole and miconazole combinations are used on wicks for several days then clotrimazole drops are used, three drops mane for ten days. The ear is reviewed and recleaned at two weeks. Approximately 20% of these cases recur months, or even years later. The patient should be warned of this possibility.

(c) *Chronic Myringitis*

This condition is characterised by a non–healing raw surface of the pars tensa and the adjacent deep canal. The aetiology is uncertain but the problem is commonly found after otological surgery or as a result of chronic otitis externa. The raw surface may present as a glistening, moist but non–inflamed area, or as a reddened, thickened or granulating site. Advanced cases may cause progressive fibrous obliteration of the deep canal, leading to severe conductive deafness. The condition is difficult to eradicate and may recur after seemingly successful treatment. The canal is cleaned thoroughly and treated as for bacterial otitis externa. Resistant cases may be cauterised with silver nitrate or trichloroacetic acid. Some persistent conditions may require surgical excision of the raw site and split–skin grafting, possibly combined with a meatoplasty to improve aeration and drying of the deep canal.

(d) *Viral Otitis Externa*

(i) Herpes Zoster

The Ramsay Hunt Syndrome is due to herpes infection of the facial nerve, presenting as a lower motor neurone facial palsy with shingles eruptions on the posterior wall of the canal and sometimes on the pinna. (See "Facial Palsy"). Management of the eruption is by local cleansing and antibacterials to prevent secondary infection.

(ii) Bullous myringitis

This condition is characterised by painful blistering confined to the tympanic membrane and deep canal. The condition is of viral aetiology – a small number of patients contract encephalitis. At presentation, blisters are seen obscuring the drum and deep canal. These are filled with serous fluid, possibly with a purplish tinge due to haemorrhage. The condition may be readily confused with acute otitis media, with serous blebs secondary to the severe middle ear infection. If in doubt, an otologist will drain the blisters and perform a myringotomy if indicated.

2.2 KERATOSIS OBTURANS

This is a cholesteatoma–like mass of keratin and cerumen located in the deep external canal. The accumulation, sometimes triggered by otitis externa, is due to failure of the normal canal–cleansing epithelial migration. It presents as an obstinate mass of debris, usually with cerumen on its superficial aspect, and may therefore resemble simple hard wax obstruction of the canal. Neglect of the condition results in the keratosis gradually expanding and eroding the skeleton of the deep canal. Destruction of the tympanic membrane and ossicular chain may follow, similar to a cholesteatoma. (Fig. 26)

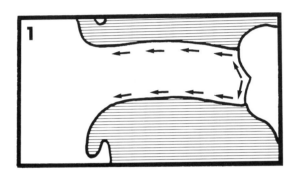

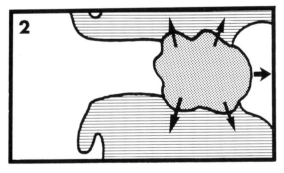

Figure 26. Keratosis obturans. The normal external auditory canal skin migrates laterally (1) removing debris, wax and keratin from the deep canal. If the mechanism fails a buildup of this debris accumulates in the deep canal causing the formation of a plug of wax and keratin which gradually expands eroding the deep canal (2).

Management

Syringing is ineffectual and sometimes complicates the situation with a secondary otitis externa. Removing the mass is frequently time–consuming and may require the use of an operating microscope and fine instrumentation. Repeat cleaning every few months may be necessary to keep the canal free of further keratin buildup.

2.3 EXTERNAL CANAL TUMOURS

2.3.1 EXOSTOSES

These benign, bony lesions occur in the deep canal and are linked to swimming in cold water. They present as sessile, bony, hard swellings antero– and postero– inferiorly in the deep meatus. Smaller, pedunculated pea–shaped lesions may be noted at twelve o'clock. The exostoses may enlarge slowly until only a very narrow cleft remains. Trapped debris frequently causes recurrent otitis externa in these cases. In troublesome cases the exostoses are removed by high–speed drilling under general anaesthesia using an operating microscope. Excellent results are usually obtained and recurrence is unlikely.

2.3.2 CARCINOMA

True canal malignancy, as opposed to deep extension from primary pinna lesions is a rare disease and is often secondary to chronic otitis media. It presents with a blood–stained foul otorrhoea and pain (as opposed to the usually painless chronic otitis media). The disease is managed by wide excision, possibly requiring total petrosectomy, followed by radiotherapy. The prognosis in larger lesions is poor due to local recurrence. Local node metastases occur early, but distant spread is rare.

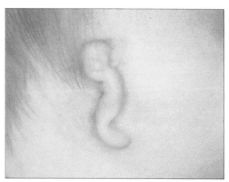

FIGURE 1.

Congenitally deformed ear with microtia and atresia of the external auditory canal. The pinna is moderately deformed, showing the typical E-deformity, but is well sited. If the problem is unilateral, surgery can be deferred indefinitely. If bilateral, bone conduction aids are fitted, followed by surgery to reconstruct the hearing mechanisms, at two years age.

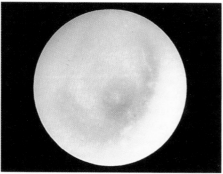

FIGURE 2.

Congenital deep canal atresia. The canal ends as a tapered blind pit. Deep to this site is an irregular bony occlusion superficial to the site of the drum. The latter is usually atrophic. The ossicular chain may be relatively well formed and mobile, or misshapen and fixed to the walls of the middle ear. A transcanal meatoplasty, myringoplasty and ossicular reconstruction may produce near normal hearing, but this surgery requires the highest otological skills.

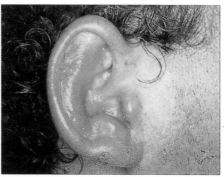

FIGURE 3.

Allergic otitis externa following topical neomycin application. The pinna has a beefy, swollen appearance. Discomfort is considerable. Clean thoroughly, including suction toilet of the canal, if possible. Apply steroid cream liberal. Resolution should be prompt.

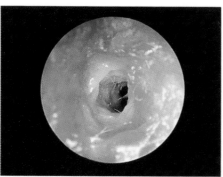

FIGURE 4.

Generalised bacterial otitis externa. Semisolid debris is seen lining the canal. Hearing may be muffled, pain may be severe. Clean by dry mopping or suction, then use a wick impregnated with broadspectrum antibiotic and steroid cream to reduce oedema and eliminate infection. Systemic antibiotics and pain relief may be required.

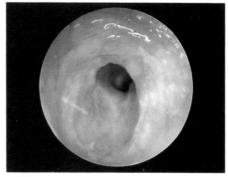

FIGURE 5.

Pseudomonal otitis externa. Typical green debris is present. Treat as per Figure 4, but if pain is severe, use a betamethasone and gentamicin ointment wick to effect optimal relief. Systemic gentamicin or ciprofloxacin may be considered.

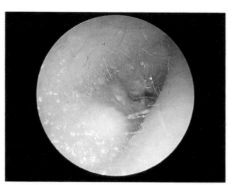

FIGURE 6.

Aural furunculosis. A small pustule is seen in the superior canal. Marked oedema may be present and pain may be extreme. The patient may be malaised, The ear will be exqisitely tender to manipulate. Manage with high dosage anti–staphylococcal antibiotics and give substantial analgesia. Use a steroid and antibiotic wick. Relief should be achieved within twenty–four hours.

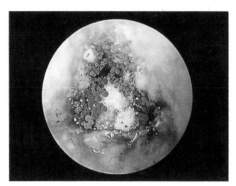

FIGURE 7.

Otomycosis due to Aspergillus nigra. The characteristic chocolate coloured spores and white mycelium fill the canal. Pruritis or discomfort may be marked. Drum ulceration and perforation are common and may be accompanied by deafness and pain. Clean meticulously by suction toilet, peeling away infected keratin from the canal wall and drum. Use topical antifungal cream, then drops for two weeks, then repeat the toilet.

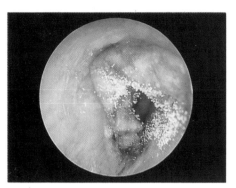

FIGURE 8.

Aspergillus flavum otomycosis. Yellow spores and mycelial debris occlude the deep canal. Treat as for A. nigra.

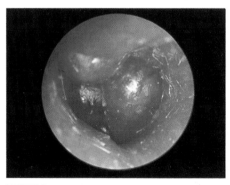

FIGURE 9.

Viral (bullous) myringitis. Severe pain precedes the formation of blebs filled with glairish fluid on the drum and deep canal. The condition closely resembles acute otitis media (Table 3.). If in doubt, treat as for AOM, provide strong pain relief if required.

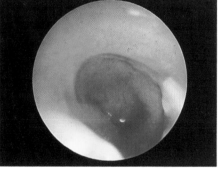

FIGURE 10.

Chronic myringitis. A velvety, raw, non–healing surface covers the deep canal and tympanic membrane. The condition is of uncertain aetiology, but occurs after repeated otitis externa, chronic otitis media and after surgery of the canal and drum. Early cases may respond to boric 5% and alcohol 70% drops, but more chronic cases require surgical clearance.

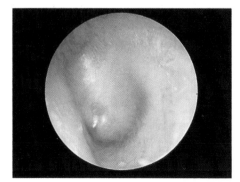

FIGURE 11.

Fibrous obliteration of the deep external canal secondary to chronic myringitis. Recurrent infection and progressive scarring have thickened the drum, producing a shortened but healed canal. A 40 decibel conductive loss results. A meatoplasty is used to dissect away the obstruction. The canal entrance is widened to promote aeration. The drum surface is grafted with fine split skin grafts.

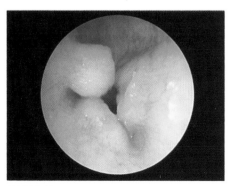

FIGURE 12.

Exostoses of the deep external canal. These are frequently associated with a history of repeated exposure to cold water (swimming, surfing etc.) Enlargement causes obstruction of the canal and accumulation of debris between the lesions and the drum. If troublesome, the exostoses are drilled away, preserving the overlying skin, via a transcanal approach.

CHAPTER 6:
FAILURE OF THE EUSTACHIAN TUBE

1. INTRODUCTION

The eustachian tube is the airway of the ear. Blockage leads to the same sequelae as bronchial obstruction, ie. collapse and filling with fluid of the distal organ. Tubal failure is the direct cause of many of the major middle ear diseases, hence the otologist's concern with regards this problem. It should be noted that the eustachian tube is essentially an outpocketing of the nasal passages. Effective tubal management will first require effective treatment of any nasal origin.

2. AETIOLOGY OF TUBAL FAILURE

2.1 IDIOPATHIC

Many cases, particularly in children, have no overt cause. The paediatric group may include cases with tubes of smaller than average diameter which require only mild oedema to cause malfunction. In aged patients, a tubal muscular failure of degenerative nature is often suspected.

2.2 INFECTION

causes oedema of the tubal epithelium with resultant blockage:

(a) Upper Respiratory Tract Infection
Acute coryza, chronic adenoiditis, sinusitis and occasionally pharyngitis are common causes, particularly in children.

(b) Otitis Media
The acute phase of acute bacterial otitis media results in oedema and therefore blockage of the eustachian tube. In those cases where drum perforation does not occur, toxins may be retained in the middle ear cleft and these may prolong the tubal oedema and obstruction.

2.3 ALLERGIC RHINITIS

and its resultant nasal mucosal oedema may extend to cause tubal obstruction.

2.4 CLEFT PALATE

cases are prone to tubal malfunction due to several reasons:

(a) Loss of the midline raphe deprives the tensor palati of its inferior anchorage during its tube–opening pulley action. (Fig. 27)

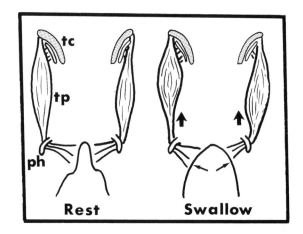

Figure 27. The aetiology of eustachian insufficiency in cleft palate cases. The cleft palate eliminates the inferior anchorage of the tensor palati in the midline raphe. During the swallowing action the tensor is deprived of anchorage inferiorly and is unable to actively open the eustachian tube by pulling down the tubal cartilage. tc: tubal cartilage; tp: tensor palati; ph: pterygoid hamulus.

(b) The tensor palati may be congenitally defective.

(c) Palatal innervation may be defective or traumatised during surgical repairs.

(d) Surgical trauma secondary to palatal repair may compromise the pulley function. Approximately 30% of cleft palate cases experience associated tubal insufficiency. Regular specialist assessments are recommended until the early adolescent years to minimise the problems of chronic tubal failure in these cases. In otherwise normal cases, the presence of a bifid uvula may indicate a submucous cleft of the palatal musculature. Failure of the tensor palati anchorage in these cases may also cause persistent tubal problems.

2.5 BAROTRAUMA

Sudden increases in extratympanic pressure may "lock" the eustachian tube and if the pressure differential becomes severe, a transudate or haemorrhage occurs. The tubal obstruction may persist up to several weeks. (See "Traumatic Ear Conditions").

2.6 CARCINOMA

of the postnasal space may present as a middle ear effusion. A unilateral serous middle ear effusion in an adult without apparent cause calls for a careful posterior rhinoscopy. People of southern Chinese ancestry are particularly prone to this malignancy.

2.7 PHYSICAL OBSTRUCTION

of the tubal orifice by a nasal septal spur is an occasional finding. The problem is corrected by a septoplasty. Temporal bone fractures may also occlude the tube.

3. SEQUELAE OF TUBAL FAILURE

3.1 MIDDLE EAR EFFUSION

3.2 COMPLICATIONS OF CHRONIC TUBAL INSUFFICIENCY

3.1 MIDDLE EAR EFFUSION

(Synonyms: Serous otitis media, Secretory otitis media, "Glue ear", Chronic mucoid otitis)

Middle ear effusions vary in consistency from serous to seromucinous, seropurulent, mucopurulent or mucoid. Many are sterile in origin and nature but others may result from persisting tubal obstruction, secondary to middle ear infections such as acute otitis media. The effusions tend to pursue a common clinical course and are considered together. Middle ear effusion is the major cause of partial deafness in children.

3.1.1 PATHOGENESIS

In sterile cases, obstruction of the tube isolates the middle ear from the atmosphere. Absorption of the air from the middle ear cleft into the surrounding tissues results in a negative middle ear pressure. As this intensifies, a serous transudate seeps into the cleft, progressively replacing the air with a honey–coloured, watery fluid. (Figs. 29(a)(b)(c)) With time, the lining mucous membranes become oedematous and the epithelium undergoes progressive metaplasia to a ciliated respiratory pattern. With this change, the effusion gradually becomes progressively mucoid. If the process begins with an acute otitis media, the air in the cleft may be resorbed or may be expelled by the buildup of seropurulent exudate secondary to the infection. Persistent blockage may continue subsequent to resolution of the infection and may lead to the later epithelial changes above.

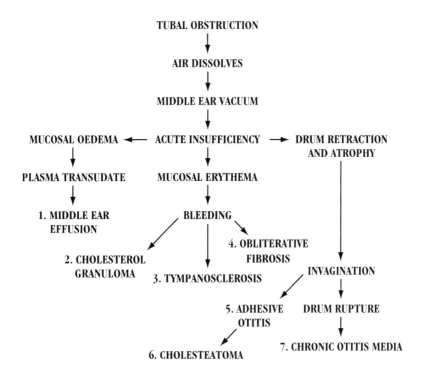

Figure 28. Results of tubal failure.

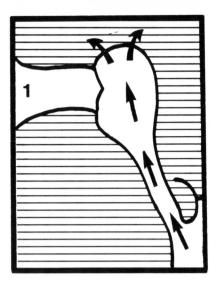

Figure 29(a).Normal eustachian tubal function. Air passes into the middle ear and mastoid air cell system and is resorbed into the surrounding bloodstream.

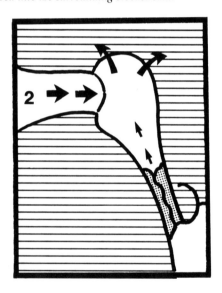

Figure 29(b).
Eustachian occlusion. The resupply of air to the middle ear is cut off with absorption of the middle ear oxygen and nitrogen. A vacuum forms and the atmospheric pressure forces the tympanic membrane medially.

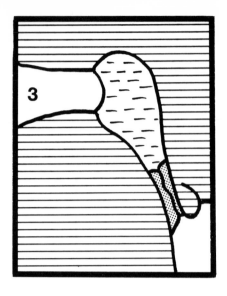

Figure 29(c). Persistent middle ear effusion results in a serous transudate into the middle ear replacing the aerated cleft with a fluid–filled cavity.

3.1.2 PRESENTATION

(a) Symptoms

(i) Pain may be present at onset, or a child may have a history of intermittent otalgia. The pain is due to tension on the drum from atmospheric pressure and is similar to that experienced when diving without equalising. The problem is silent in many cases, but eustachian insufficiency ranks with acute otitis media as a major cause of earache in children.

(ii) Discharge may occur during an initiating or previous otitis media.

(iii) Deafness is present but subtle, usually 15–20 decibels. This is sufficient to cause mild but noticeable hearing problems in children. Adults note a blockage in the affected ear.

(iv) Tinnitus, (described by adults), is initially squeaking or bubbling in nature. With complete filling of the ear by effusion the ringing of physiological tinnitus may become more noticeable to the patient. Children rarely complain of tinnitus.

(v) Vertigo or unsteadiness is noted on occasion. The cause is uncertain. Infants may appear clumsy on their feet.

(b) Signs

Detection of a middle ear effusion requires a good auriscope light and a clean canal. As the ear passes through a spectrum of changes as the glue ear forms, some experience is required for accurate diagnosis. Drum changes:

(i) A red and retracted membrane denotes acute insufficiency. If unilateral, compare the affected ear with the unaffected side.

(ii) Bubbles, coalescing into fluid levels, result from the initial serous transudate forming in the middle ear. (These may be present also in resolving cases but these cases are less inflamed).

(iii) A straw–coloured tympanic membrane, in sterile cases, is caused by the middle ear completely filling with the yellowish–brown serous transudate.

(iv) With time, as the mucosa of the middle ear undergoes metaplasia to form goblet cells, the serous transudate becomes a mucoid exudate. The drum takes on a grey or waxy discolouration with vessels radiating from the tip of the handle of the malleus – "cartwheel vasculature".

In cases due to otitis media, the acute phase passes leaving a grey membrane with prominent radiating vessels.

3.1.3 INVESTIGATION

(a) ENT history and examination

particular attention is directed towards possible causative conditions in the upper respiratory tract. Check for adenoid infection or hypertrophy.

(b) Radiology

is used to assess the upper respiratory tract. Sinus and lateral postnasal space films help identify sinus infection and adenoid hypertrophy and carcinoma of the postnasal space in adults.

(c) Tympanometry

is a valuable screening test to detect effusions (flat curve – Type B) and tubal insufficiency (negative range peaks – Type C. See Chapter I). The tensor tympani and stapedius reflexes are absent with effusion. Suspicious tympanograms warrant referral if a good view of the drum cannot be obtained.

(d) Audiometry

has limited value in middle ear effusions, as the hearing is usually reduced by only 15–20 decibels and losses of this extent are frequently found in children due to lack of attention or poor testing circumstances (Fig. 30)

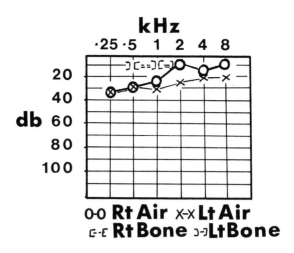

Figure 30. Mild conductive deafness. The twenty–five to thirty decibel conductive losses are typical of the mild losses encountered in middle ear effusions.

3.1.4 TREATMENT

The management of middle ear effusions remains controversial due to the multiplicity of factors involved in its aetiology. In particular, the role of adenoidectomy remains uncertain. It should be noted that accurate assessment of adenoiditis in the child is frequently impossible, however many cases are clearly secondary to an adenoid cause and removal of the adenoids is well warranted in these cases.

(a) Conservative

As many cases are directly related to nasal sepsis and as significant numbers of these infections are relatively covert, the nose is routinely managed medically to minimise any risk of a nasal origin of the tubal insufficiency. Antihistamines, often combined with phenylephrine or pseudephedrine, are used to reduce nasal and tubal oedema and to minimise nasal secretion. Nasal sympathomimetic sprays may be used over short periods to help clear infected debris by either physiological or nose–blowing manoeuvres. The role of the Valsalva manoeuvre is uncertain. Cases of minor obstruction may be helped by forced insufflation of the ears whilst pinching the nose or whilst using one of a variety of commercial devices to promote this manoeuvre. Local sepsis in the nose and throat is usually due to streptococcus pneumoniae, haemophilus or moraxella. Treat any infection with amoxycillin/clavulanic acid or cefaclor.

(b) Surgical

Failed conservative treatment (after approximately 4–6 weeks), complications, or urgency in a particular case (eg. necessity to fly) may indicate surgical intervention. This treats the upper respiratory tract cause and ventilates the middle ear.

(i) Upper respiratory tract:
Adenoidectomy (Fig. 31) may minimise further postnasal space infection.

Sinus drainage or washouts may eliminate sepsis due to sinusitis.

Tonsillectomy. This is frequently undertaken in conjunction with the above when tonsillitis is a problem in its own right, or may be undertaken in selected cases where persistent tonsillar infection is considered contributory to the middle ear effusions.

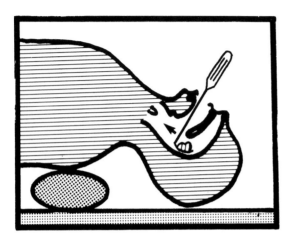

Figure 31. Adenoidectomy. The patient is laid in the supine position and the adenoidal mass is curetted from the postnasal space via the mouth.

(ii) Ear Drainage and Ventilation :

Technique. The effusion is drained via a radial myringotomy, usually in the anteroinferior quadrant of the pars tensa. In most cases, a small ventilation tube ("grommet") will be used. The role of the tube is to simply maintain a hole in the pars tensa, thus providing a temporary tubal bypass. Standard Teflon, silicone or polythene tubes usually last about 8-12 months before spontaneous extrusion occurs. The precise cause of the extrusion remains uncertain but is probably related to a combination of factors, including the normal epithelial migration across the drum surface and low grade foreign body reactions. Prior to extrusion, the tube is frequently noted to acquire a "cuff" of dead skin. Upon extrusion, the tube may fall out completely, or may lodge in canal wax, to be carried laterally by the canal epithelial migration. Cases in which ventilation tubes are inserted are reviewed regularly until the tubes have fully extruded.

Complications of Ventilation Tubes

Recurrent cases may require repeat insertions using longer lasting models.

Fifteen percent of cases require repeat procedures.

Otorrhoea through the tube occurs in 5-10% of cases and is due to otitis media as a result of pathogens entering the middle ear from either the

eustachian tube or the ventilation tube itself. The former often follows an upper respiratory tract infection, whereas the latter usually results from water entering the ear via the ventilation tube. To prevent the latter, custom-made silicone ear plugs are usually fitted for bathing or swimming. Episodes of otorrhoea are managed as for perforated acute otitis media (amoxycillin/clavulanic acid, cefaclor, antibiotic drops). Persistent cases are managed with gentamicin drops, which are particularly effective if a granulation has formed on or near the ventilation tube. These granulations are easily removed with a fine sucker.

Chronic mastoiditis or cholesterol granuloma may be unmasked by the insertion of a ventilation tube. They present as intractable mucopurulent otorrhoea from the time of insertion and will require a simple mastoidectomy to clear the disease.

Drum atrophy. Small atrophic scars result at the tube insertion site in some cases but are generally not troublesome. Repeated insertions, together with the intractable tubal insufficiency, may result in more significant drum atrophy.

3.2 COMPLICATIONS OF CHRONIC TUBAL INSUFFICIENCY

3.2.1 ADHESIVE OTITIS

Gradual collapse of the tympanic membrane into the middle ear is a not infrequent result of chronic tubal insufficiency. Atrophy and collapse of the drum usually begin in the posterosuperior quadrant. Anterior pars tensa atrophy is less common. The drum atelectasis is accompanied by adhesions as a result of inflammation or haemorrhage. Membrane collapse may be followed by avascular necrosis of the ossicular chain, sometimes with fixation of the malleus or stapes by tympanosclerosis.

Presentation: The history is that of occasional otalgia due to episodes of acute insufficiency, without otorrhoea. Deafness is gradually progressive, up to 60-70 decibels. On examination, the drum is noted to be collapsed medially in the posterosuperior quadrant of the posterior half. The ossicular chain may be skeletonised by the collapse, and necrosis of the incus or stapes may be observed. Tympanosclerosis is often present.

Management in early cases is to prevent further tubal insufficiency. Long-term grommets are more frequently used in these cases. Severely damaged cases undergo tympanoplasty using cartilage-stiffened grafts to reinforce the drum and microprostheses to repair the ossicles. Cases of intractable tubal failure may require a hearing aid to regain hearing.

3.2.2 TYMPANOSCLEROSIS

Pathology. Tympanosclerosis is a deposit of calcific material in the middle ear. Its pathogenesis is uncertain, but it usually occurs after middle ear inflammation and probably haemorrhage. The calcification is usually noted as chalky patches in the tympanic membrane itself due to thin plaques in the middle layer of the drum. Less often, masses of the chalky material occur in the middle ear, sometimes fixing the ossicular chain.

Presentation. Tympanosclerosis is usually a coincidental finding in the tympanic membrane. In advanced cases, deafness appears gradually and is sometimes severe, often with a past history of chronic middle ear disease.

3.2.3 CHOLESTEROL GRANULOMA

Pathogenesis. Bleeding into the middle ear cleft and mastoid air cells system may result in cholesterol crystal formation secondary to breakdown of the blood. The crystals may excite a foreign body reaction which causes excessive mucous secretion from the ear.

Presentation. The condition is unusual and may present with a "blue ear drum" or idiopathic haemotympanum. Myringotomy produces a copious mucoid drainage which persists despite grommet insertion.

Management. Remove surgically via a cortical mastoidectomy.

3.2.4 CHRONIC SUPPURATIVE OTITIS MEDIA.

Chronic negative pressure on the drum results in weakening and atrophy, leading to breakdown and perforation. A proportion of cases of non–healing drum perforations are therefore due to tubal insufficiency. (See Middle Ear Infections).

3.2.5 CHOLESTEATOMA

Invagination of an atrophied drum secondary to chronic tubal insufficiency may form a sac extending through the middle ear into the mastoid air cell system. The sac of keratinising stratified squamous epithelium is not a neoplasm but has the potential to destroy the ear. (See Middle Ear Infections).

PICTORIAL ESSAY
FAILURE OF THE EUSTACHIAN TUBE

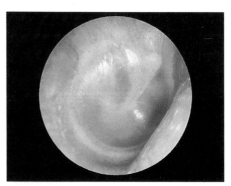

FIGURE 1.

Normal tympanic membrane. The drum has a shallow loudspeaker shape and a pearly transluscent lustre. The "light reflex" is seen in the anteroinferior quadrant. The long process of the incus is seen behind the posterosuperior drum.

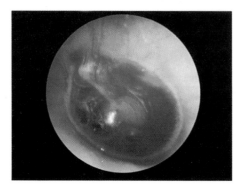

FIGURE 2.

Acute barotrauma subsequent to diving during an influenza episode. Haemorrhagic fluid and bubbles are seen behind the drum. Pain at onset is usual, the ear feels blocked and deaf. The condition resolves spontaneously, usually in one to two weeks. If distressing, a temporary mini-tube insertion is performed under topical anaesthesia for immediate relief.

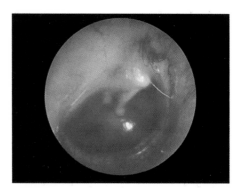

FIGURE 3.

Serous middle ear effusion secondary to tubal obstruction. Gradual resorption of middle ear air results in suction on the lining of the cleft. A honey-coloured transudate has resulted. Mild conductive deafness is present. Compare the drum appearance with figure 1.

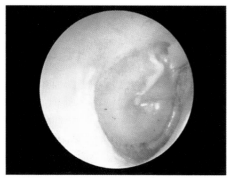

FIGURE 4.

Purulent effusion secondary to AOM. The acute phase has passed and the inflammation has resolved, leaving the drum discoloured by the purulent effusion in the middle ear. Retained bacterial toxins may perpetuate tubal oedema and insufficiency.

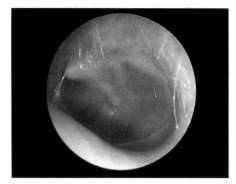

FIGURE 5.

Chronic mucoid otitis media. Prolongued middle ear effusion has been followed by gradual metaplasia of the lining of the cleft. Goblet cells have proliferated, resulting in increased mucus content of the effusion, which may achieve a viscid consistency ("glue ear"). Compared with figure 1, the drum has a dead gray appearance. Ventilation produces rapid reversal to the normal appearance.

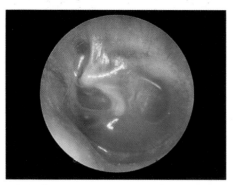

FIGURE 6.

Resolving seropurulent effusion. Tubal recovery has allowed partial re-aeration. Bubbles and fluid levels are seen behind the drum. Inflammation is absent, as the middle ear pressure has returned to normal levels. Total resolution is imminent.

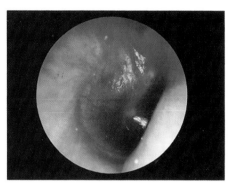

FIGURE 7.

Idiopathic haemotympanum. Past bleeding into the middle ear as a result of acute insufficiency has produced a blackish discolouration of the drum. Longstanding cases may be associated with the formation of cholesterol granuloma. Ventilation tube insertion in the latter cases may result in prolonged mucoid otorrhoea. Surgical clearance of the mastoid may be required.

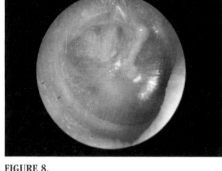

FIGURE 8.

Early adhesive otitis. Prolonged tubal failure and negative middle ear pressure gradually weaken the pars tensa. Stretching and collapse typically begin in the posterosuperior quadrant of the drum, which is draped over the long process of the incus in this case. The middle ear is aerated.

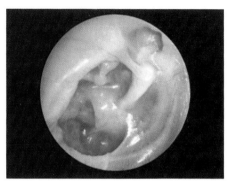

FIGURE 9.

Severe adhesive otitis. Marked drum atrophy and collapse cover the middle ear structures with a transparent film of squamous epithelium. The long process of the incus is partially necrosed. A chronic effusion is present. The appearance is often confused with a large drum perforation.

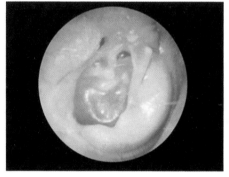

FIGURE 10.

Advanced adhesive otitis. Gross posterior drum collapse is accompanied by necrosis of the long process of the incus. The anterior drum is grossly tympanosclerotic and deposits of this are also seen adjacent to the stapes. A chronic mucoid effusion is probably present. A severe conductive loss is present. Tympanoplasty is unlikely to effectively restore hearing.

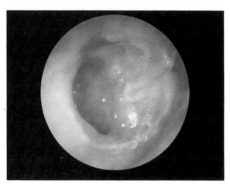

FIGURE 11.

Chronic otitis media secondary to tubal insufficiency. Gross drum collapse has resulted in a large posterior perforation. The head of the stapes is seen in the posterosuperior middle ear. The incus has necrosed and the handle of the malleus is retracted. A myringoplasty and ossicular chain reconstruction are indicated. Drum stiffening by fine cartilage grafts will be needed to prevent recollapse.

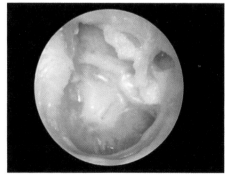

FIGURE 12.

Advanced destruction of the middle ear. Total drum collapse has resulted in complete elimination of the middle ear cleft. The remnants of the malleus are seen anterosuperiorly. The incus and stapes have necrosed. The footplate of the stapes is seen just below the horizontal facial nerve. Cholesteatoma formation has occurred in the attic and is actively eroding the superior scutum. Fine squamous epithelium completely lines the site. Restoration of hearing will be difficult and will depend on the viability of the tubal function.

CHAPTER 7:
MIDDLE EAR INFECTIONS

CLASSIFICATION

1. BACTERIAL

1.1 ACUTE OTITIS MEDIA
1.2 CHRONIC OTITIS MEDIA

2. CHOLESTEATOMA

1.1 ACUTE OTITIS MEDIA

Acute otitis media (AOM) is one of the common childhood illnesses. Virtually no family goes untouched. Presentation is usually during winter or spring. The typical sufferer is a febrile three to five year old, mouthbreathing, with a discharging nose. A wet cough may be present and the child may be from a lower socio-economic background. The family may be well-known to the attending family physician for its history of respiratory tract infections or ear disease in other children.

The epidemiological pattern is the result of the middle ear's relationship to the nose. Embryologically and functionally, the middle ear is an outpocket of the post-nasal space. Infants are prone to multiple viral infections in the nose, maximal during the first years of contact with the general community. These predispose to bacterial nasal, then ear infections. Hitherto, upper respiratory tract infections and otitis media peaked in incidence at four to six years – the years of kindergarten and primary school. Now, with increasing numbers of mothers in the workforce, group childcare is common at earlier ages and therefore the disease patterns are increasing in the younger age group.

The viral upper respiratory tract infections are maximal from late autumn to early spring; AOM follows after a short delay. Generally, the specialist sees the problem later still, after the disease has become repetitive or has resisted initial therapy in the general practice situation.

The otitis media sufferer may display a range of related problems. Chronic nasal congestion and purulent rhinorrhoea are typical of enlarged and infected adenoids. Sinusitis may also be present. Asthma, presenting as a loose, perhaps wheezy cough, is commonly present and is often exacerbated by inhalation of infected material from the infected adenoid pad. Tonsillitis may be present, usually in conjunction with Streptococcus pyogenes. Adenotonsillar enlargement, combined with asthma, may give a typical "puffing billy" or "goldfish" syndrome.

The effect on the family of the miserable child afflicted with the above should not be underestimated. The mother may be fatigued from late nights tending a sick child and the father may feel excluded from the mother-child relationship or be subject to emotional outbursts from the stressed mother. Resultant child abuse is not unknown. Increased pressure on the practitioner for an early cure may result from the family stress.

After repeated AOM, or after a severe episode, lingering deafness or otorrhoea may suggest presence of a non-healing drum perforation, characteristic of chronic otitis media (COM).

1.1.1 AETIOLOGY OF ACUTE OTITIS MEDIA

(a) Anatomy

The middle ear chamber is normally a sterile air-filled chamber enclosed by rigid bony walls except for the tympanic membrane on the lateral aspect. The only entrance is the eustachian tube, extending from the postnasal space next to the adenoid pad. The cleft is lined with simple squamous epithelium. Ciliary epithelium is found mainly in the eustachian orifice and tube but only sporadically elsewhere in the middle ear. Ciliary action is thus efficient in the eustachian tube but less so elsewhere in the cleft.

(b) Pathogenesis of AOM.

In acute infections, soiling of the chamber by pathological bacteria usually involves, in order of frequency, Streptococcus pneumoniae, Haemophilus influenzae, Moraxella cartarrhalis and some Streptococcus pyogenes and Staphylococcus aureus. The process often begins with a viral infection in the nose which results in mucosal damage. Impaired ciliary action results in retention in the nose of mucus and the protein-rich effusion from the damaged surface. Superinfection by the above pathogens follows. Forced insufflation of the middle ear by sneezing or nose blowing may instil bacteria into the ear, or these may enter by normal ear ventilation via the eustachian tube. The middle ear mucosa poorly resists infection. Inflammation, then effusion into the cleft, rapidly

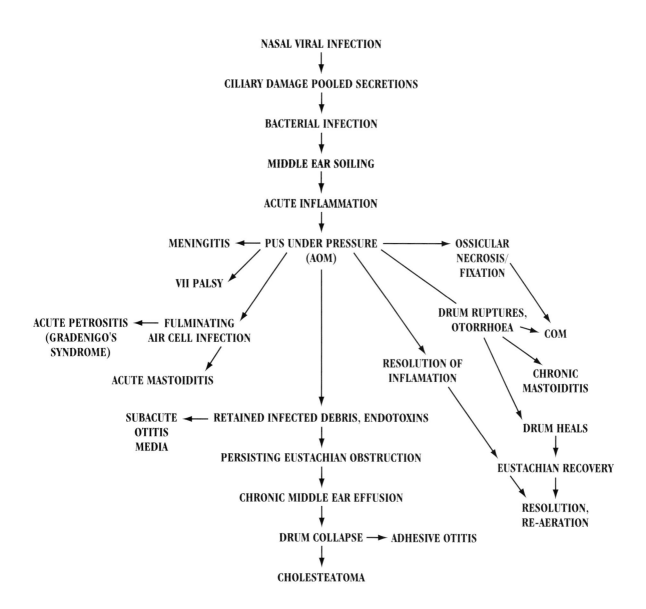

Figure 32. Pathogenesis of otitis media and its sequelae

produces pus under pressure when the eustachian tube (minimum diameter 1mm.) closes due to oedema. Pressure builds up on the drum, stretching the collagenous middle layer. Blebs of serous effusion may form on the inflamed drum, or the squamous epithelium may rupture giving a macerated appearance. The collagenous layer may hold firm, or may rupture releasing a seropurulent, perhaps bloodstained discharge through the external auditory canal. (Fig. 32)

The rupture releases the pressure and drains endotoxins from the middle ear cleft. Recovery after drum perforation is frequently rapid as a result. The perforation, usually less than 1mm. diameter, closes within days, leaving little trace behind. In non-ruptured cases, the inflammation abates, usually after seven to ten days. Oedema within the cleft resolves and tubal function recommences. Reaeration occurs over two to four weeks. In some cases, tubal recovery is delayed by persistent oedema resulting in mucopurulent middle ear effusions for extended periods.

1.1.2 PRESENTATION OF ACUTE OTITIS MEDIA
HISTORY

The presenting complaint of AOM is usually otalgia, frequently severe and of brief duration. Children may indulge in head banging, or demonstrate other distress, but in a large minority of paediatric cases, the problem may be asymptomatic. The infected ear is partially deaf. Otorrhoea is commonly an early sign and in children, often the first manifestation. Adults may describe blockage plus popping or gurgling-type tinnitus accompanied by agonising pain if the ear is forcibly or auto–inflated. The patient commonly feels unwell. Febrile episodes are common in children, sometimes with febrile convulsions.

FINDINGS

Examination of the infected ear may be difficult. Wax or debris in the external meatus may prevent an adequate view of the drum. A child may be fractious, may resist canal cleaning, or may wriggle during otoscopy. Clean the ear by gentle mopping and avoid suction in children.

In AOM a range of findings may be observed. At the onset, the drum is red; mixed air and purulent effusion are seen behind the drum. This phase passes rapidly as the middle ear fills with purulent effusion. The inflamed drum then begins to bulge laterally. Perforation, resolution, or persistent effusion follow.

If the drum is perforated, seropurulent or bloodstained otorrhoea fills the canal. A pinhole perforation may be noted discharging pulsatile debris. Otorrhoea is a frequent presentation of AOM in children. Spontaneous closure usually occurs in a few days. The canal then dries up, the drum loses its erythema and the purulent debris behind the drum progressively aerates as the eustachian tubal function returns. The drum may return to a normal appearance in two weeks.

Without perforation, resolution may be more protracted. The erythema fades leaving a distended but non–inflamed drum which may then aerate back to the normal appearance or alternatively, a slow change to the dead grey waxy appearance of chronic glue ear may be noted as the effusion gradually becomes more mucoid. Radial or "cartwheel" vessels may be noted on the drum. In some cases, a low grade infection perpetuates a yellow and inflamed drum appearance.

RELATED PATHOLOGY

Disease may be found in the nose and throat. Mouthbreathing, mucopurulent rhinorrhoea and a large pair of tonsils may suggest adenoid hypertrophy. If adenotonsillar enlargement is present, inquire regarding snoring, restlessness or apnoea whilst the child sleeps, to determine any nocturnal upper airway obstruction. Check for general failure to thrive, and other evidence of poor general health and hygiene. A sallow, pasty, fatigued countenance is typical of nocturnal airways difficulty.

1.1.3 INVESTIGATIONS

(a) Microinspection.
Suction toilet and inspection of the tympanic membrane under the operating microscope yield considerable information.

(b) Bacteriology.
Due to the rapidity of the clinical course of AOM, cultures are not normally performed. In repetitious cases they are more valuable to determine the identity of the pathogen and the appropriate management. Bacteriology of the nose and any otorrhoea is essential if any of the complications below are present.

(c) Tympanometry
may confirm a middle ear effusion in doubtful cases but is not advisable in the acute phase due to discomfort, or when otorrhoea is present from a ruptured drum. It is a valuable tool to check for post–AOM glue ear at four weeks post–infection.

(d) Audiology
is used after AOM if persisting deafness is suspected. Precise audiology in children is possible only in optimal conditions and should be undertaken by a skilled audiologist.

(e) Radiology
may demonstrate a causative upper respiratory tract

condition, especially adenoid hypertrophy or sinus disease.

1.1.4. TREATMENT OF ACUTE OTITIS MEDIA

An AOM patient may be unwell and in pain. Prompt, effective treatment is called for. Medical management primarily requires antibiotic therapy appropriate to the likely pathogen. Amoxycillin/clavulanic acid or cefaclor are the drugs of choice as the likely pathogens are almost all sensitive to these agents. If allergy to both these agents is present, use cotrimoxazole or erythromycin. Use maximal dosage for age, q.i.d. for two days, then continue for seven to ten days at the normal dosage. Provide adequate analgesia. Treat any antecedent upper respiratory tract infection with topical nasal decongestant sprays (Drixine, Otrivine) and systemic sympathomimetic-antihistamine combinations (Demazin, Dimetapp or Actifed). These will clear the nose and promote eustachian tube recovery.

If otorrhoea has begun, clean the canal thoroughly and sterilise with topical antibiotics. Use aqueous-based drops, rather than an oil-based preparation. A wick may be preferable to absorb the discharge and maintain the antibiotic in situ. Replace wicks on a one to two day basis depending on the degree of otorrhoea. Generally, the discharge will take about five to seven days to clear.

In cases of severe pain, the acute phase may benefit from myringotomy and possibly grommet insertion. Acute myringotomy (Fig. 33) should be confined to skilled, practised hands because of the risk of damage to the middle and inner ear contents. It is performed to release pressure, therefore reducing the pain of the stretched drum. If expertise is not available, eg in remote areas, intravenous antibiotics and adequate pain relief are a satisfactory alternative. Grommet insertion under topical anaesthesia provides rapid relief for adults and older children and promotes rapid recovery. The drum is initially desensitised using one of a variety of agents. Concentrated Phenol, Bonain's solution (Phenol, menthol and cocaine) or more recently, Emlar Cream are used. In children, the milder agents (Bonain's or Emlar) are preferred. Phenol acts faster but causes transient slight stinging which is not tolerated by many children. Insertion of a ventilation tube in the acute phase will be followed by a period of otorrhoea. Treat as for perforated AOM. The grommet is removed in adults after one to two months. In children, the tube is left until spontaneous extrusion takes place.

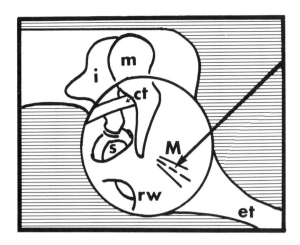

Figure 33. Acute myringotomy. Drainage of the middle ear is undertaken via the anteroinferior quadrant. This avoids the vital structures in the other areas of the middle ear. m: malleus; i: incus; s: stapes; ct: chorda tympani; rw: round window; et: eustachian tube; M: myringotomy site.

1.1.5 RECURRENT AOM

Repeated attacks usually occur in infants, frequently complicating upper respiratory tract infections. A six to eight week trial of phenoxymethylpenicillin and Demazin is worthwhile, using a b.d. normal dose for age. Refractory cases require surgery. Ventilation tubes are used to abolish the severe otalgia typical of the condition. The grommets may produce a profound improvement in the family environment, as the sufferer no longer regularly wakes the household in the middle of the night. This scenario alone explains much of the popularity of ventilation tubes.

Concurrent management of the upper respiratory tract may minimise further episodes by eliminating a causative nasal condition. Adenoidectomy, antral washouts and possibly tonsillectomy may be required.

Recently an ill-advised trend has arisen, opposing the use of antibiotic treatment. This trend ignores the frequency of major complications in the pre-antibiotic era when mastoidectomy wards were the norm in major paediatric hospitals. Patients who are concerned about the use of antibiotics should be reassured of their safety, and also warned of the risk of major complications in untreated cases.

1.1.6 COMPLICATIONS OF ACUTE OTITIS MEDIA

Although middle ear infections are a common childhood malady which are readily and effectively managed in the primary care situation, it should be noted that these conditions are capable of major complications (Fig. 34). In the past they were a leading cause of childhood morbidity and mortality. Fulminating infections may cause diffuse acute mastoiditis throughout the air cell system. Particularly in the young, the infection may break through the mastoid cortical bone leading to a subperiostial abscess. This presents as an erythematous swelling posterosuperior to the pinna. If fluctuant, incision and drainage with a cortical mastoidectomy is required.

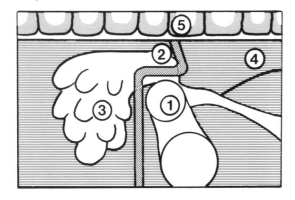

Figure 34.   Complications of acute otitis media.
1. Chronic drum perforation.
2. Facial palsy.
3. Acute mastoiditis.
4. Petrositis.
5. Central nervous system infections.

Cases without abscess formation are managed with high dose intravenous antibiotics (the same drugs as in AOM) plus drainage of the middle ear by a grommet insertion. Extension to the petrous apex cells may cause a sixth nerve palsy as it crosses the apex and a resultant lateral rectus palsy. This, plus retro-orbital pain (involvement of the fifth at the same site) and ipsilateral otorrhoea are the signs of Gradenigo's Syndrome.

Facial palsy is a not uncommon result of acute middle ear infection and is an otological emergency. Drain the ear by a myringotomy and grommet insertion, then treat with high doses of the appropriate antibiotics, plus steroids if the palsy is severe. Recovery is usual if treatment is prompt and appropriate. Immediate referral of all facial palsies to an otologist is recommended to avoid delays in cases such as this. Meningitis and intracranial infections were a common problem in the pre-antibiotic era but now are less often seen. Suspect an otological origin in unexplained bacterial meningitis.

Permanent deafness may follow the acute episode. A minor conductive loss due to mucosal fibrosis is an occasional finding. More severe losses are the norm in chronic otitis media. Sensorineural losses are occasionally seen after AOM.

1.2 CHRONIC OTITIS MEDIA (COM)

(a) Definition

Chronic otitis media refers to those ears in which the eardrum has a chronic non-healing perforation. The perforation may or may not be associated with ossicular fixation or necrosis, middle ear infection, tympanosclerosis or mastoiditis. (Fig. 35)

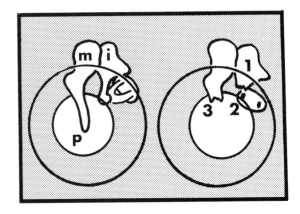

Figure 35.   Pathology of chronic otitis media. This condition is characterised by a chronic perforation of the tympanic membrane (p). Ossicular damage may result. Most common is necrosis of the long process of the incus (1), secondly, necrosis of the stapes superstructure (2) and lastly necrosis of the handle of the malleus (3). m: malleus; i: incus.

(b) Aetiology

A chronic perforation in the drum may arise from several causes. Overwhelming infection may result from either a virulent bacteria such as in scarlet fever (haemolytic streptococcus), or alternatively, in debilitated patients, particularly after measles or malnutrition. Repeated episodes of otitis media as a result of chronic upper respiratory tract infections may also cause progressive weakening and rupture of the drum. Chronic tubal insufficiency can also weaken the drum, progressing to atrophy and perforation.

1.2.1 PATHOGENESIS

If a permanent perforation of the drum forms due to the above causes, the middle ear mucosa, being poorly disease-resistant, is then prone to infection entering from the external meatus, particularly when waterborne. Repeated acute or chronic episodes lead to mucosal fibrosis and a change of epithelial quality to a ciliated secretory respiratory pattern. Further infections will lead to ossicular fixation or necrosis. Extension of infection into the mastoid air cell system produces chronic mucosal infection, osteitis and resultant non-remitting otorrhoea due to chronic mastoiditis.

1.2.3 PRESENTATION

Pain is unusual and is frequently associated with acute superinfection of the exposed middle ear. Most cases are deaf, the extent being due to the position and size of the drum perforation. Deafness tends to be worse in cases with posterior perforations than in those with anterior patterns. Deafness will be more severe in cases of fixation or destruction of the ossicles or during acute infection. Otorrhoea is a common finding and is secondary to bacterial contamination of the middle ear from either the external meatus or via the eustachian tube. Tinnitus is present in many cases, particularly during otorrhoea (crackling or popping) or may result in chronic cases from longstanding ototoxin exposure. On examination a purulent mucoid otorrhoea may be noted in the external canal. Adherent, dry debris and foul khaki-coloured discharge are frequently seen. Granulations and chronic myringitis may be present in the deep canal. The middle ear mucosa may be clean and gleaming if non-inflamed, or alternatively oedematous and polypoidal. Use of a tuning fork will demonstrate a conductive deafness (See Chapter 1). If chronic mastoiditis is present, a pulsatile otorrhoea may be observed.

1.2.3 INVESTIGATIONS

(a) Microinspection

The status of the middle ear cleft, mastoid, ossicular chain and hearing are frequently assessed by this manoeuvre alone.

(b) Bacteriology

This is more relevant in COM than AOM, due to the greater diversity of pathogens involved. Bacteriology before surgical intervention is particularly useful to select the appropriate pre- and post-surgical treatment.

(c) Audiology

This will show a conductive loss of variable extent. A large drum defect or ossicular pathology will produce conductive losses of greater than 40 decibels. Some sensorineural deafness is common in longstanding chronic perforations and needs to be accurately assessed as it will mitigate restoration of hearing by tympanoplasty.

1.2.4 COMPLICATIONS OF CHRONIC OTITIS MEDIA

These are similar to those of acute bacterial otitis media and are usually a result of an acute superinfection.

1.2.5 MANAGEMENT

(a) Conservative

Non-surgical treatment is undertaken to sterilise an infected situation either to eliminate the active infection or as a preparation for surgery. Local and systemic measures are used. Local management includes meticulous cleaning of the debris in the external canal and middle ear. Fine suction toilet under microscopy is optimal, otherwise use dry mopping with wool carriers under direct vision. The canal and middle ear are then managed with antibiotic and steroid combinations. Betamethasone and gentamicin are valuable if pseudomonal infections are present, particularly when resistant to neomycin. Systemic broad spectrum antibiotics are used to reduce active ear infection, including ciprofloxacin for acute or persistent pseudomonal infections.

(b) Surgical Management

The surgical management of chronic otitis media has a threefold aim:

(i) Repair of the tympanic membrane: myringoplasty

(ii) Repair of the ossicular chain: ossiculoplasty

(iii) Eradication of mastoiditis if present: cortical mastoidectomy

(Tympanoplasty is a looser term, covering both membrane and ossicular reconstruction. See Chapter 8 – "Middle Ear Surgery").

2. CHOLESTEATOMA

Cholesteatoma is a sac–like invagination of the tympanic membrane epithelium into the middle ear. Once formed, the sac tends to expand and destroy adjacent structures. It is the covert danger of middle ear disease because of its tendency to potentially fatal complications due to its proximity to the central nervous system. Nonetheless, it is not a neoplasm. Its aetiology is complex but many are due to chronic eustachian tubal failure with resultant weakening and indrawing of the tympanic membrane. (Fig. 36)

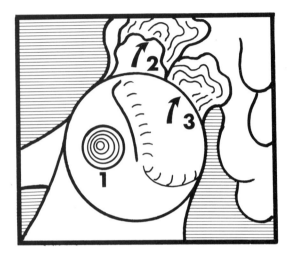

Figure 36.   Patterns of cholesteatoma.
1. Congenital middle ear cysts.
2. Attic cholesteatoma.
3. Pars tensa cholesteatoma.

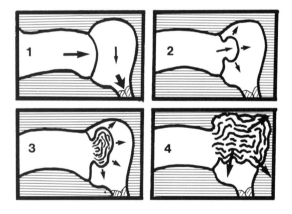

Figure 37.   Genesis of pars tensa and attic cholesteatoma. Many of these lesions have an origin in chronic tubal insufficiency. This produces chronic negative pressure in the middle ear, gradual weakening of the tympanic membrane, invagination, then loss of the self cleaning mechanism, collection of debris, infection, gradual expansion and erosion of surrounding structures.

2.1 PRESENTATION

Pain is present only in acute flare–ups of the condition. Otorrhoea in these cases is foul–smelling. Bloodstaining may be present from granulation tissue protruding into the external meatus. Deafness is common and is secondary to destruction or fixation of the ossicular chain and tympanic membrane. A crackling or bubbling type tinnitus may be present. The onset of vertigo is ominous and tends to indicate extension into the inner ear. Facial palsy is not uncommon.

On examination a foul discharge is encountered in the external canal, possibly with granulations being visible on the tympanic membrane. The latter spell trouble and cases of granulation on the membrane should be referred for specialist opinion. The entrance to the cholesteatomatous sac is found either above the handle of the malleus at twelve o'clock on the tympanic membrane or in the posterosuperior quadrant. Pearly white sheets of keratin may be evident protruding through the perforation and a conductive deafness is noted on tuning fork testing. This is confirmed on audiometry. Radiology may show defects due to erosion by the sac.

2.2 MANAGEMENT

(a) Conservative

Surgery in these cases is mandatory unless the patient is unfit for anaesthesia. Conservative management is similar to that used in chronic suppurative otitis media and is employed to stabilise acute flare–ups of the condition and also as a preparation for surgery.

(b) Surgical

The surgery of cholesteatoma is controversial, with two main techniques employed:

(i) Radical or modified radical mastoidectomy.

(ii) Combined approach tympanoplasty.

2.3 COMPLICATIONS OF CHOLESTEATOMA

The complications of cholesteatoma vary according to the direction of expansion of the sac (Fig. 38). The most common extensions are into the attic, then posteriorly into the mastoid.

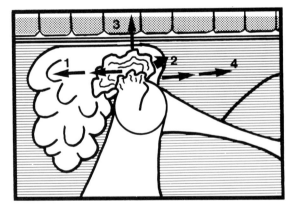

Figure 38.   Spread of cholesteatoma.

1. Posteriorly.
2. Medially.
3. Superiorly.
4. Anteriorly.

(a) Medial extension (Fig 39)

(i) Ossicular chain and tympanic membrane destruction result in conductive deafness up to 60 decibels. In many cases, sound may be transmitted through the sac itself, producing an apparently good hearing situation, albeit an unstable one.

(ii) Facial paralysis results from infection or invasion of the seventh nerve.

(iii) Further medial extension causes breaching of the bony otic capsule, then suppurative labyrinthitis. The patient presents with gross rotatory vertigo and nausea, roaring tinnitus and profound sensorineural deafness. Meningitis may follow and urgent surgery with central nervous system antibiotic cover is required. Ear swabs and CSF (if meningismus is present) are taken to identify the pathogens prior to surgery.

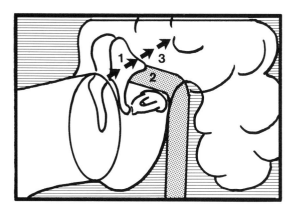

Figure 39. Complications of the medial spread of cholesteatoma.
1. Ossicular necrosis.
2. Facial palsy.
3. Fistula of the otic capsule and bacterial labyrinthitis.

(b) Superior extension (Fig 40)

(i) Extension superiorly breaches the tympanic plate, resulting in an extradural abscess.

(ii) Meningitis or subdural abscess occur if the dura necroses and perforates.

(iii) Cerebritis and temporal lobe abscess follow extension of infection into the adjacent cerebral hemisphere. The patient will show general signs of a space-occupying lesion or the local signs of a temporal lobe lesion including:

* Speech difficulties

* Aberrations of vision due to involvement of the optic radiation.

* Hallucinations of taste and smell.

* Emergency neurosurgical involvement is indicated in all these conditions.

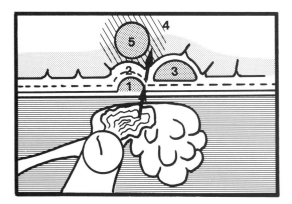

Fig 40. Complications of the superior spread of cholesteatoma.
1. Extradural abscess.
2. Meningitis.
3. Subdural abscess.
4. Temporal lobe cerebritis.
5. Temporal lobe abscess.

(c) Posterior extension (Fig 41)

(i) Acute mastoiditis and superficial abscesses present similarly to those cases due to acute otitis media. Cholesteatoma tends to occur in an older age group.

(ii) Lateral sinus thrombophlebitis may result in septicaemia or disseminated abscesses. Retrograde thrombosis may destroy the function of the arachnoid granulations, causing otitic hydrocephalus or alternatively, cavernous sinus thrombosis.

(iii) Invasion of the posterior fossa results in the range of intracranial complications referred to in (b)(iii) above. Cerebellar abscesses present with coarse nystagmus, dysdiadokokineses, aberrant reflexes and unsteadiness, the patient falling to the side of the lesion.

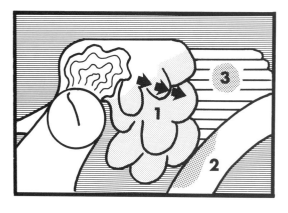

Figure 41. Complications of the posterior spread of cholesteatoma.
1. Acute mastoiditis, superficial or deep cervical abscesses.
2. Lateral sinus thrombosis, septic distal emboli and abscess formation.
3. Central nervous system infections, cerebellar abscess.

(d) Anterior extension

Forward extension is rare, but the resultant petrositis may cause Gradenigo's Syndrome: trigeminal distribution pain and lateral rectus palsy (due to V and VI involvement at the petrous apex) together with ipsilateral otorrhoea. Evacuation of the petrous apex cholesteatoma is a considerable surgical exercise.

(e) Iatrogenic Complications

Facial paralysis occurs due to the nerve being camouflaged by the disease process and surgical nerve damage in this situation is not rare. "Dead ears" may result from surgical manoeuvres at a fistula site, from breaching the otic capsule with a drill, or from trauma to the ossicular chain. Radical mastoidectomy cavities may cause the patient a lifetime of otorrhoea.

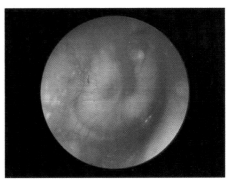

FIGURE 1.

Early acute otitis media (AOM). The middle ear is diffusely infected with Str. Pneumoniae, H. Influenzae, or M. Catarrhalis and has filled with purulent exudate. The drum is bulging laterally under pressure. Pain is severe, fever and malaise are present. Acute myringotomy in skilled hands may give considerable relief.

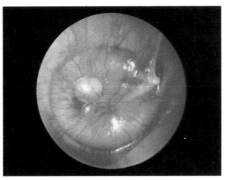

FIGURE 2.

AOM, early bleb formation. The drum is injected and under pressure. Serous fluid forced through the drum forms a small vescicle on the posterior pars tensa.

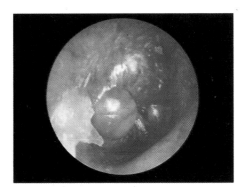

FIGURE 3.

AOM, advanced bleb formation. The appearance may be indistinguishable from viral myringitis. Drum perforation is imminent and will result in reduction of discomfort and general toxicity.

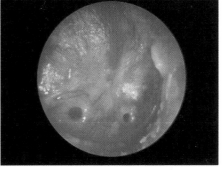

FIGURE 4.

Perforated AOM. Small dual perforations are seen in the pars tensa. Seropurulent, mucopurulent, or bloody otorrhoea may be present. The perforations are frequently minute and may not be seen. The defects close within a few days, followed by a rapid resolution phase. Healing may be complete within two weeks.

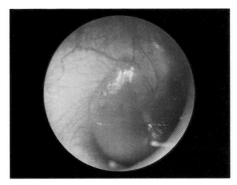

FIGURE 5.

AOM, early resolution phase. The tympanic membrane is intact and still distended. The inflammatory phase has passed. Purulent fluid is seen behind the pars tensa, with a collection of semi–solid yellow debris inferiorly.

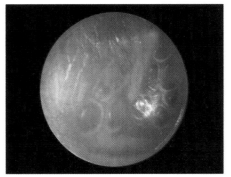

FIGURE 6.

Advanced resolution phase of AOM. Bubbles behind the drum herald the return of tubal function and reaeration of the middle ear cleft. Hearing should return to normal.

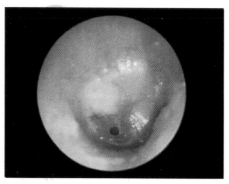

FIGURE 7.

Chronic otitis media (COM). A small non-healing perforation is evident in the posteroinferior pars tensa. The drum is sclerosed, but the ossicular chain is probably intact and mobile. Hearing loss should be minimal. A small plug of fibrous tissue will suffice to repair the defect.

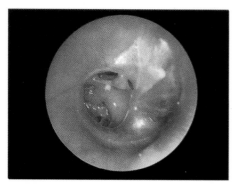

FIGURE 8.

A larger defect in the posterior pars tensa. The middle ear mucosa is healthy, but the defect site is more audiologically sensitive and the loss from the lesion may be twenty-five to thirty decibels. A limited repair, using temporalis fascia or perichondrium should restore function completely.

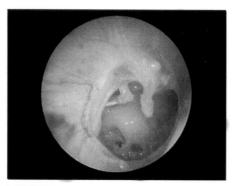

FIGURE 9.

Total loss of the drum secondary to scarlet fever. The middle ear mucosa has recovered to the normal state. The malleus handle, long process of the incus, stapedius tendon and stapes superstructure can be seen in the upper middle ear. A forty decibel loss is likely, more if ossicular fixation has occurred. Myringoplasty will require more extensive grafting. A homograft membrane may be used to repair defects of this extent.

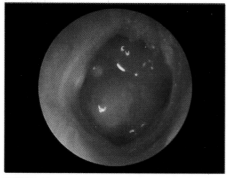

FIGURE 10.

Total drum loss and severe middle ear damage. The mucosa is inflamed, thickened and chronically discharging. The malleus and incus are necrosed. The stapes is seen posterosuperiorly. Myringoplasty, columellar ossiculoplasty and, possibly, cortical mastoidectomy will be required to seal the defect and restore hearing. The audiological prognosis is guarded, due to the extent of pathology.

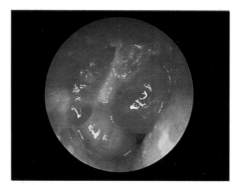

FIGURE 11.

A grossly diseased middle ear. Profuse granulation formation obscures details of the drum and other anatomy. Cholesteatoma cannot be excluded. Full exploration of the middle ear and mastoid will be required to clear the disease. Poor audiological prognosis.

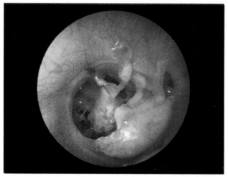

FIGURE 12.

Longstanding COM complicated by marked drum and middle ear tympanosclerosis formation. The anteroinferior drum remnant is stiffened by the marked calcification. Tympanosclerosis deposits are seen posterior to the handle of the malleus. These are fixing the stapes superstructure. Attic fixation of the malleus and incus is probable. A sixty decibel loss is present. The pathology will require staged surgery to recover function, possibly incorporating stapedectomy and subsequent ossiculoplasty.

PICTORIAL ESSAY
CHOLESTEATOMA

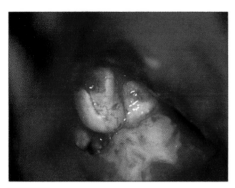

FIGURE 1.

Cholesteatomatous sac in the middle ear. Surgeon's view during exploration of the mastoid. A pearly sac is seen in the attic space just above the head of the stapes, seen lower right. Despite the name, the lesion is a simple sac of keratinising stratified squamous epithelium, histologically identical with the tympanic membrane.

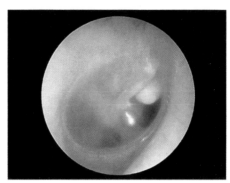

FIGURE 2.

Congenital cholesteatoma. A tiny cyst is seen in typical location, just anterior to the handle of the malleus. The cyst may remain unchanged for long periods, or growth may accelerate, especially after episodes of AOM. Removal by a transcanal approach should eliminate the problem, with retention of normal hearing.

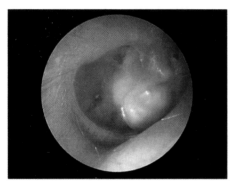

FIGURE 3.

A larger variant of figure 2. The cyst extends deep to the handle of the malleus and touches on the stapes superstructure. Removal may be difficult, particularly if a diagnostic myringotomy has caused attachment to the drum or malleus handle. Removal may require a postaural approach, possibly with removal of the malleus handle or part of the drum, if the cyst is adherent. Ossicular involvement may require an ossiculoplasty, but in the absence of other middle ear pathology, the results of such surgery should be good.

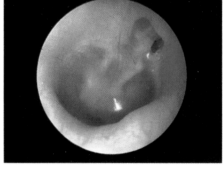

FIGURE 4.

Attic retraction pocket. A small, clean pocket, as seen just above the handle of the malleus, is a relatively common finding. These are kept clear of debris by the normal external canal epithelial migration. Failure of the flow of epithelium out of the pocket is the trigger which activates the formation of attic cholesteatoma.

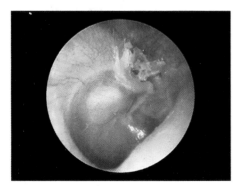

FIGURE 5.

Attic cholesteatoma. Failure of the self–cleaning mechanism has resulted in formation of a keratin plug in the pocket. The latter has deepened to form a sac which is evident behind the posterosuperior pars tensa and deep to the drum just anterior to the malleus. The ear has remained free of infection. Hearing may remain good, due to transmission of sound through the sac itself.

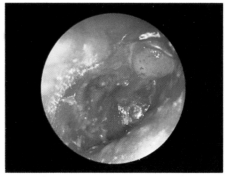

FIGURE 6.

Attic polyp. A vascular polyp is seen at the site of the pars flaccida. Foul or bloodstained otorrhoea commonly accompanies this scenario. Granulations on or near the drum usually require specialist evaluation to exclude the presence of cholesteatomatous otitis media.

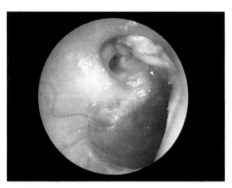

FIGURE 7.

Active attic cholesteatoma. A large chronically infected attic sac is present. Necrotic keratin is seen protruding from the sac orifice. A middle ear effusion is present. Chronic otorrhoea, deafness and foul odour are troublesome. Surgical clearance is required to abolish the symptoms, restore function and to avoid the major complications associated with the disease.

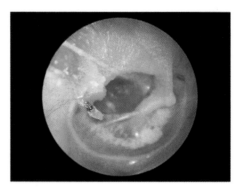

FIGURE 8.

Pre-cholesteatomatous severe adhesive otitis media. A marked retraction of the postero-superior pars tensa has resulted in necrosis of the long process of the incus and the stapes superstructure. The retraction has hitherto remained clear of keratin, but the epithelial flow is now failing. Early debris accumulation is seen at ten o'clock. Progressive buildup will lead to infection and granulations, then extension of the sac deeper into the middle ear.

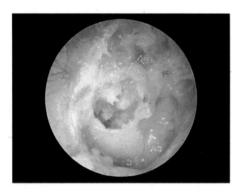

FIGURE 9.

Established pars tensa cholesteatoma. A large sac is seen, filled with keratin. Extension behind the lower drum is present. The lesion extends superiorly into the attic, then posteriorly into the mastoid. These patterns are more difficult to clear surgically and require specific drum stiffening techniques to prevent recurrence.

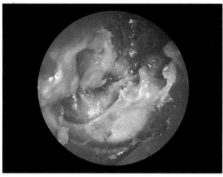

FIGURE 10.

Extensive combined pars tensa and attic distribution cholesteatoma. Marked erosion of the attic wall superior to the drum has occurred. Similar erosive disease is likely elsewhere in the middle ear cleft. The facial nerve, otic capsule and the central nervous system are particularly at risk. Early surgical intervention is desirable.

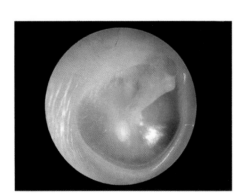

FIGURE 11.

Inclusion cholesteatoma. A small cyst is seen in the posteroinferior pars tensa, secondary to a prior myringotomy. Observation alone may suffice, as the lesion may spontaneously extrude. Enlargement can be countered by simple removal under topical or local anaesthesia.

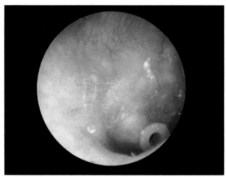

FIGURE 12.

Inclusion cholesteatoma secondary to the insertion of a ventilation tube. A cyst is seen just posterior to the tube. Transcanal removal, after elevation of a tympanomeatal flap, plus tube removal and a limited myringoplasty should eliminate the problem.

INTRODUCTION

Middle ear surgery is performed on microscopic structures under conditions of difficult access to a frequently bleeding operating field. Infection, tubal insufficiency and other difficulties must be anticipated and avoided. To meet these challenges, the operating microscope was originally developed, in Sweden, specifically for otology. Middle ear surgery includes reconstructive procedures, grouped under tympanoplasty, plus other procedures required for removal of infection, cholesteatoma, or other disease. Considered separately below is the unique problem of otosclerosis and its management by stapedectomy.

CLASSIFICATION OF MIDDLE EAR SURGERY

1. DRUM REPAIR:

1.1 MYRINGOPLASTY

2. OSSICULAR CHAIN RECONSTRUCTION:

2.1 OSSICULOPLASTY

3. MASTOID SURGERY:

3.1 CORTICAL/SIMPLE MASTOIDECTOMY

3.2 RADICAL MASTOIDECTOMY

3.3 MODIFIED RADICAL MASTOIDECTOMY

3.4 ATTICOTOMY

3.5 COMBINED APPROACH TYMPANOPLASTY

3.6 MASTOIDECTOMY RECONSTRUCTION

4. SURGERY FOR OTOSCLEROSIS:

4.1 FENESTRATION

4.2 STAPEDECTOMY

1.1 MYRINGOPLASTY

The repair of a drum defect requires closure of the defect by a free graft which will eventually have air on each side. Free grafts require vascular ingrowth and therefore stability to avoid shearing off this capillary supply. Drum repairs therefore require three phases to meet this requirement: site preparation, graft siting, and graft support and immobili-

sation. One of several tissues can be used, including autogenous, temporalis fascia, perichondrium, periosteum or external canal skin. Homograft or heterograft tissues such as dura, tympanic membrane transplants or preserved animal tissues have also been used in the past, although these have now fallen out of favour. A transcanal or postaural approach may be used. The edge of the drum defect is first detached to create a circumferential raw surface from which vascular ingrowth will originate. The posterior eardrum and adjacent canal skin are elevated and reflected forwards as a tympanomeatal flap. The middle ear is then filled with absorbable gelatin sponge to provide medial support for the graft. The latter is then positioned immediately deep to the drum defect and the tympanomeatal flap is then laid back onto the graft. The external canal is then lined with non–adherent dressings and is lightly packed. The graft is thus stabilised between the gelatin sponge and the external canal dressings to ensure revascularisation (Fig. 42)

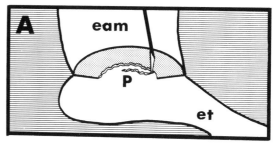

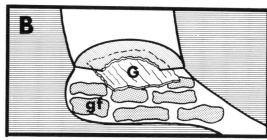

Figure 42.   Myringoplasty technique.

A.The drum perforation (P) is de–edged to create a vascular origin to revascularise the drum graft. eam: external auditory meatus; et: eustachian tube.

B.The middle ear is filled with supportive Gelfoam pledgets which are sited immediately deep to the drum. The graft is then fixed between the Gelfoam support and light dressing placed in the external canal. Success rates are approximately ninety per cent. G: graft; gf: Gelfoam.

Myringoplasty in expert hands should provide a better than 90% success rate. Some population groups (eg. children, some indigenous races, poor socioeconomic groups) may suffer a higher complication rate. Extensive defects and persistent eustachian tubal malfunction also carry higher risks.

2.1 OSSICULOPLASTY

Ossicular chain reconstruction is essentially micro–orthopaedics, however, in its final position the reconstruction will be placed in the air–filled chamber of the middle ear with minimal attachment to surrounding tissues. These reconstructions may be undertaken simultaneously with a myringoplasty or at a second stage to allow graft healing and therefore greater stability of the tympanic membrane and surrounding tissues. The long process of the incus is the site most commonly damaged, followed by stapes superstructure necrosis, then destruction of the malleus handle (Fig. 43).

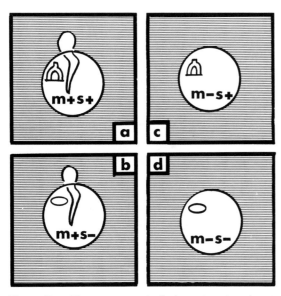

Figure 43.   The common ossiculoplasty situations (Austin classification).
a. Both the malleus handle and the stapes superstructure are present. Absence of the incus is the most common ossicular necrosis situation.
b. Absence of the stapes superstructure in addition to the incus.
c. Absence of the malleus and the incus.
d. Absence of the malleus, incus and stapes superstructure.m: malleus; s: stapes superstructure.

In cases of minimal pathology, microprostheses are fitted between the malleus handle and the stapes or footplate. These procedures are termed assembly techniques and provide a stable and usually successful reconstruction. In more advanced destruction, when the malleus handle is absent, a "columellar" prosthesis is placed between the tympanic membrane and the stapes head or footplate (Fig 44).

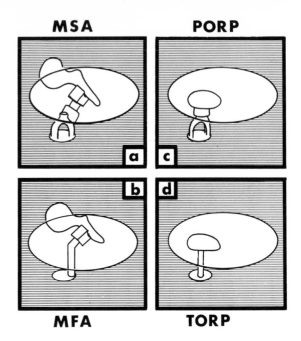

Figure 44.   Ossiculoplasty techniques. If the malleus handle is present, assembly techniques can be used to reconstruct the ossicular chain between the malleus handle and the stapes superstructure (a): the malleus stapes assembly (MSA). If the malleus handle is present but the stapes superstructure is absent, a malleus footplate assembly (MFA) is used (b). If the malleus handle is absent a partial ossicular replacement prosthesis (PORP) or short columella is used between the tympanic membrane and the superstructure of the stapes (c). If all the ossicular structures are gone, a long columella or total ossicular replacement prosthesis (TORP) is used to connect the tympanic membrane and the footplate of the stapes (d).

These columellar techniques are both successful and popular, but may be complicated by prosthetic displacement or extrusion of biomaterials through the tympanic membrane. Ossicular reconstructions can be performed using autograft or homograft ossicles, reshaped for the purpose, but ossicle techniques are now being superseded by specialised microprostheses manufactured from selected biomaterials. Older materials such as polyethylene have given way to prostheses made of hydroxylapatite. Calcium phosphate is sintered at 2000°C, producing a non–soluble, bioactive ceramic which produces little tissue reaction. In minimally damaged situations, ossiculoplasties are successful in up to 90% of cases. In more severely damaged cases, the success rate will fall according to the pathology present.

3. MASTOID SURGERY

3.1 CORTICAL MASTOIDECTOMY

Cortical, simple, or Schwarz's mastoidectomy, is undertaken for non-cholesteatomatous disease, such as acute or chronic mastoiditis, or cholesterol granuloma. The procedure is designed to clear the mastoid air cells system posterior to the external canal, but not entering the canal, the middle ear or the attic. The mastoid is exposed via an endaural or postaural incision and the soft tissues are reflected off the bony process. The latter is then cleared by a high-speed drill and continuous irrigation. Particular care is taken to avoid damage to the lateral sinus posteriorly, the dura superiorly and the facial nerve and external canal lying anteriorly. The air cells are cleared progressively until the confines of the mastoid are skeletonised. (Fig. 45) The technique should have few complications but care must be taken in infants to avoid the very superficial facial nerve present in these cases. In expert hands the procedures are usually successful. Reconstruction of the middle ear may be combined with a cortical mastoidectomy if necessary.

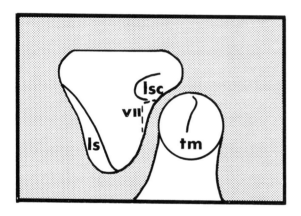

Figure 45. Cortical mastoidectomy. The mastoid air cell system is exenterated, clearing the cells between the dura above, the lateral sinus behind and the external canal anteriorly. lsc: lateral semicircular canal; VII: facial nerve; ls: lateral sinus; tm: tympanic membrane.

3.2 RADICAL MASTOIDECTOMY

The presence of active cholesteatoma in the middle ear is usually a mandatory indication for surgery because of its tendency to cause major complications. The disease may be managed by "open" or "closed" surgery. The traditional "open" techniques of managing cholesteatoma have been to regard the lesion as being tumour-like and therefore to excise as far as possible all those tissues with which the cholesteatoma has come in contact. In radical mastoidectomy, a cortical mastoidectomy-type procedure is undertaken and then is extended to remove the posterior and superior external canal wall, together with the diseased ossicular chain and all, or part of, the tympanic membrane if involved with disease. A meatoplasty is undertaken to expose the resultant cavity to ready access from the external canal for the purpose of postoperative cavity cleaning. (Figs. 46 (a)(b))

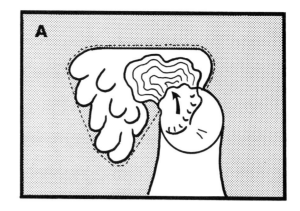

Figure 46(a). Radical mastoidectomy. This technique applies tumour principals to excision of the cholesteatoma where the drum is badly damaged. The dotted line indicates the extent of excision.

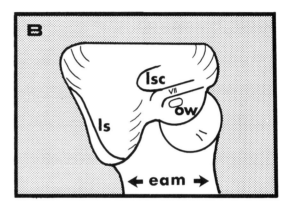

Figure 46(b). Radical mastoidectomy site. The drum is partially absent and a large cavity is present above and behind the site of the membrane. The external canal is widened by means of a meatoplasty. ow: oval window; eam: external auditory meatus; ls: lateral sinus; lsc: lateral semicircular canal.

3.3 MODIFIED RADICAL MASTOIDECTOMY

If the tympanic membrane is intact and healthy, this will be retained, forming a modified radical mastoidectomy. The open cavity thus created measures approximately 2-3cm across. This is left open via the external canal and in many cases, the cavity will re-epithelialise with squamous epithelium and become clear of infection, although periodic cleaning is required, usually on a six to twelve monthly basis.

Regrettably, in a proportion of cases, persistent infection will result from an open tympanic membrane or from accumulation of debris and infection in the bowl of the cavity itself. This may require revision surgery or mastoidectomy reconstruction. In cases of radical mastoidectomy, tympanoplasty is not undertaken but in many cases of modified radical mastoidectomy, the eardrum is sealed and ossiculoplasty may be performed. The latter will frequently give excellent results. (Figs. 47(a)(b))

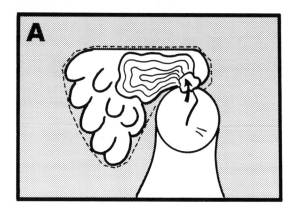

Figure 47(a). Modified radical mastoidectomy. In this modification of the radical procedure, the tympanic membrane is spared but the open cavity is otherwise created similar to the radical procedure.

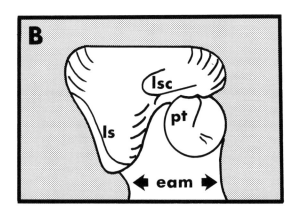

Figure 47(b). Extent of the modified radical mastoidectomy procedure. The tympanic membrane remains intact. lsc: lateral semicircular canal; ls: lateral sinus; eam: external auditory meatus; pt: pars tensa.

3.4 ATTICOTOMY

is a very limited open technique similar to a modified radical mastoidectomy. Only the attic area is opened to the external canal, forming a mini-cavity. Fewer complications result, but the procedure is confined to cases of limited disease.

3.5 COMBINED APPROACH TYMPANOPLASTY

The incidence of problem cavities secondary to the open surgery above led to the development of "closed" procedures to avoid these complications. Combined approach tympanoplasty, which allows access to the disease via both the external canal and the mastoid site during surgery, is designed to leave the ear with a normal external canal after the surgery. The procedure is an extension of the cortical mastoidectomy. The epitympanum is cleared of ossicles and disease from behind and laterally and the middle ear is entered by removal of the bone between the facial nerve and the rim of the tympanic membrane: posterior tympanotomy. By these approaches, the middle ear can be inspected to permit clearance of cholesteatoma whilst retaining the external canal

and avoiding an open cavity. (Figs. 48(a)(b))

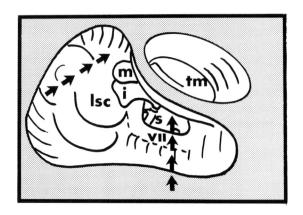

Figure 48(a). Combined approach tympanoplasty. The procedure eliminates cholesteatoma by a posterior approach to the attic and middle ear. A posterior tympanotomy created just lateral to the facial nerve allows good access to the posterior middle ear itself. m: malleus; i: incus; lsc: lateral semicircular canal; s: stapes; VII: facial nerve; tm: tympanic membrane.

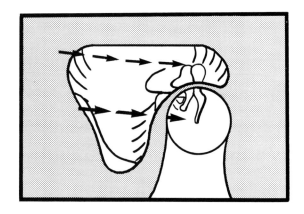

Figure 48(b). Lateral aspect of the combined approach tympanoplasty.

The procedure is normally undertaken in two stages: at the first stage the disease is cleared and the tympanic membrane is repaired. Twelve months later, the ear is re-inspected to ensure the absence of residual disease which may have been missed at the first stage. This occurs in 20% of cases. Removal of the tiny cysts of residual disease, if present at the second stage, is not usually a problem. Reconstruction of the ossicular chain may be undertaken at the first stage or delayed until the second stage if severe disease is present at initial surgery. Results of ossiculoplasty are comparable with the results from non-cholesteatomatous surgery. Whilst combined approach tympanoplasty is technically more difficult than open procedures and requires two stages, it avoids the ongoing problem of a suppurating open cavity and is more effective in restoring hearing. The patient can enjoy water sports and does not require routine cavity cleaning.

3.6 MASTOIDECTOMY RECONSTRUCTION

In those cases of radical or modified radical mastoidectomy in which persistent otorrhoea or other cavity complications are a problem, reconstruction of the external canal is possible to rehabilitate the ear. Canal wall restoration is undertaken by either obliterating the mastoid cavity with solid tissue such as bone chips, ceramic granules or cement, or alternatively, by reconstructing the canal wall. Cartilage or hydroxylapatite ceramic implants are used for the latter. In expert hands, otorrhoea is usually abolished, but reconstruction of the hearing in these badly damaged cases is more difficult. In modified radical mastoidectomy cases, where the tympanic membrane remains largely intact, hearing results are often good. In badly damaged radical cases, the results are poorer.

4. OTOSCLEROSIS

PATHOLOGY

Otosclerosis is an aberrant proliferation of immature bone, developing on and around the stapes footplate. The problem is a congenital abnormality and usually develops in the third decade of life. The bone thickening fixes the stapes footplate, preventing sound vibration from passing into the cochlea. The condition is not a neoplasm and has no other clinical significance other than its effect on hearing. (Figs. 49(a)(b))

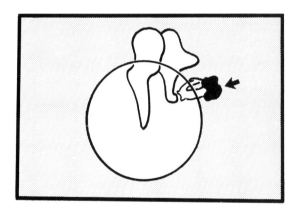

Figure 49(a). Otosclerosis. The ossicular chain is fixed by a proliferation of immature bone on the footplate of the stapes.

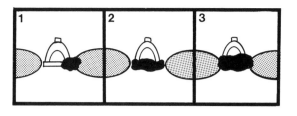

Figure 49(b). Varieties of otosclerotic fixation of the stapes footplate.

1. Focal fixation.

2. "Biscuit" formation.

3. Obliterative fixation.

HISTORY

The patient notices a gradually worsening deafness, usually beginning in the third or fourth decade. Females are more frequently affected and there may be a strong family history of deafness, although the disease may jump generations. The deafness may be bilateral or unilateral and typically worsens during pregnancy. Tinnitus may be noted due to either inner ear degenerative effects of the disease or due to the normal physiological tinnitus becoming more noticeable. There is no history of vertigo, discharge or pain. On examination, the tympanic membrane appears normal. Tuning fork tests will show a conductive deafness pattern (See Chapter 1): the Weber is felt in the deaf ear and the affected ear is Rinne negative.

INVESTIGATIONS

Pure tone audiology shows unilateral or bilateral conductive deafness. The loss is frequently confined to the lower frequencies, between 250-2000 cycles per second. There may be a superimposed sensorineural deafness with a slight loss at 2000 cycles per second. The latter, if present, is termed a "Carhart's notch". In unilateral cases tympanometry may show a flattened normal (Type A) curve when compared with the normal ear. With progression of the disease, in some cases, severe sensorineural deafness may become a distressing feature of the otosclerosis. The cause is uncertain, but the sensorineural losses may progress to profound or subtotal deafness. (Fig. 50)

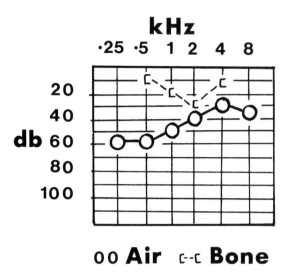

kHz

Figure 50. Pure tone audiometry in otosclerosis. A conductive deafness is present. A small depression in the sensorineural reserves is seen at two thousand cycles per second. This is termed a Carhart's notch and is typical of otosclerosis.

MANAGEMENT

Otosclerosis responds well to hearing aids in the early to moderate phase and an aid may be preferred to surgery. The latter, however, is the preferred form of treatment. Otosclerosis was originally managed by fenestration surgery. This was similar to a modified radical mastoidectomy but included creation of a surgical fistula in the lateral semicircular canal. The surgery was effective in many cases, but was difficult, frequently complicated and often unrewarding.

Stapedectomy was introduced in 1958. The stapes superstructure is gently removed in whole or part, under a local or general anaesthesia. The fixed footplate is then perforated by micro-instrumentation or by power drilling, and a tiny micropiston of Teflon, stainless steel or composite construction is used to replace the stapes. The piston has a hook which is fitted around the long process of the incus and crimped to grasp the incus securely. The piston itself leads through the small perforation in the footplate into the cochlea. The results of stapedectomy are excellent, with good results being obtained in over 90% of cases. (Fig. 51)

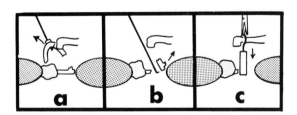

Figure 51. Stapedectomy. a. The stapes superstructure is removed after initial division of the incudostapedial joint and stapedius tendon. b. A small area of the footplate is removed by micro-instrumentation or with a fine drill. c.

The partially removed stapes is replaced by a micro-piston crimped around the long process of the incus. Excellent results are the norm from this surgery.

A tiny percentage will, however, suffer a "dead ear", but this should be a rare occurrence. Postoperative transient vertigo is common, although usually not severe. The patient is instructed to rest quietly for approximately two weeks postoperatively and to avoid severe exercise or work for a further month. In the postoperative period, the patient often notices echoing or crackling sounds which herald the return of hearing. Complete return of hearing takes about six to eight weeks, at which time complete restoration of hearing up to the sensorineural reserves is commonly achieved. Late complications from stapedectomy are unusual but include perilymph fistula, where a minute leakage of perilymph occurs at the operation site. These patients may require re-exploration and sealing of the problem as a surgical emergency. If managed promptly, hearing may be completely salvaged.

PICTORIAL ESSAY
MIDDLE EAR SURGERY

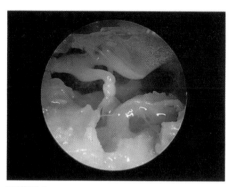

FIGURE 1.

Normal middle ear cleft. The handle of the malleus is seen attached to the undersurface of the loudspeaker-shaped tympanic membrane above. The incus is seen to the left, articulating with the head of the stapes, centrally. The facial nerve is seen as a pink line just behind the stapes superstructure. Ossicular fixation may be due to otosclerosis at the footplate of the stapes, or to incus or malleus fixation in the attic. Ossicular necrosis most often affects the long process of the incus, then the stapes superstructure and the malleus handle.

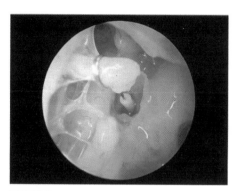

FIGURE 2.

Stapedectomy. The stapes superstructure has been removed, and a small area of footplate has been removed to permit entry into the cochlea. A micropiston comprising a cylindrical Teflon shaft and a platinum ribbon "shepherd's crook" has been implanted to restore transmission. The ribbon is crimped around the long process of the incus (top left). The Teflon shaft passes into the cochlea. Excellent results are expected in over ninety percent of cases.

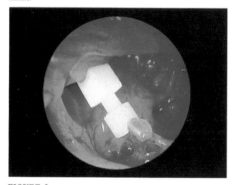

FIGURE 3.

Malleus-stapes assembly. Only the incus is absent- the most common ossiculoplasty situation (Austin Group A). A "Spanner" prosthesis is placed between the handle of the malleus (top left) and the stapes superstructure. In this best risk group good results are obtained in over eighty percent. The head of the prosthesis is dense hydroxylapatite ceramic. The shaft is Teflon.

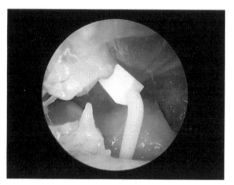

FIGURE 4.

Malleus-footplate assembly. The incus and stapes superstructure are absent (Group B). A long "Spanner" is sited between the malleus handle and the footplate of the stapes (below, obscured by the facial nerve). Tubal insufficiency and other major pathology may be present, thus success rates are less – about seventy percent.

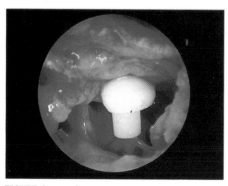

FIGURE 5.

Partial ossicular replacement prosthesis (PORP). Used when the incus and malleus are absent (Group C) or when the malleus is unsuitable for a malleus-stapes assembly. The PORP columella transmits sound from the drum itself to the stapes head. The hydroxylapatite head has excellent biocompatibility. Complications include displacement, fixation and extrusion. Success rates in the Group C situation are about sixty percent.

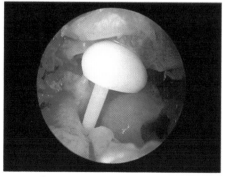

FIGURE 6.

Total ossicular replacement prosthesis (TORP). These implants are used in the worst case situation, when the malleus, incus and stapes superstructure are all absent or damaged (Group D). The sound passes from the drum through the hydroxylapatite head and the Teflon shaft of the prosthesis, to the stapes footplate and thence into the cochlea. The prostheses are prone to similar complications to the PORPs, plus a greater risk of tubal insufficiency. As a result, Group D success rates are approximately fifty-five percent.

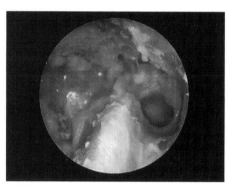

FIGURE 7.

Radical mastoidectomy. The entire middle ear cleft has been exenterated to remove the threat of cholesteatoma. A large defect is seen in the drum (right). The cavity has become badly infected and will require ongoing toilet to minimise discomfort. The ear is severely deaf.

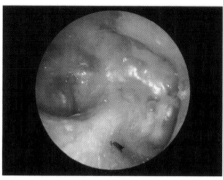

FIGURE 8.

Modified radical mastoidectomy. Similar surgery to Figure 7 has been undertaken, but the drum has been preserved and the middle ear is sealed off. The cavity site has healed well and self-cleaning epithelial flow has been re-established. Hearing levels may be good. This is an optimal result for open cavity surgery.

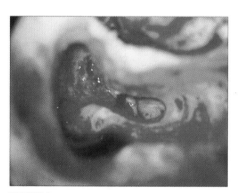

FIGURE 9.

Intact canal wall mastoidectomy and posterior tympanotomy (combined approach tympanoplasty). The mastoid is cleared of disease, then the attic and middle ear are approached from behind. Seen is a right ear, during surgery, with the external canal above. The stapes is seen centrally, through the posterior tympanotomy. The "closed cavity" procedure permits removal of cholesteatoma or other diseases, whilst preserving the skeletal supports of the drum and the external canal, thus avoiding the above open cavity situation.

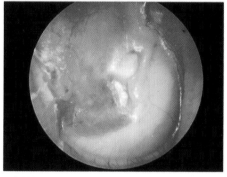

FIGURE 10.

Pars tensa cholesteatoma managed by intact canal wall surgery. A large area of collapse has been excised and the drum grafted. The head of a "Spanner" is seen engaging the malleus handle. Hearing results are within satisfactory levels. Grafts incorporating finely shaven sheets of cartilage are required in this situation, to prevent drum recollapse. Closed cavity procedures require a second stage at twelve months, to check for residual disease.

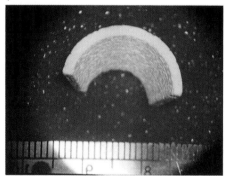

FIGURE 11.

Grote porous hydroxylapatite ceramic canal wall replacement implant. Open cavities are prone to chronic infection, discomfort, foul odour and other distressing symptoms. Grote implants and custom-designed vascular flaps enable the external canal to be completely rebuilt to rehabilitate the middle ear.

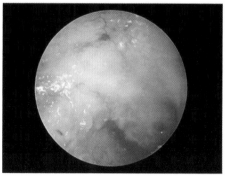

FIGURE 12.

Mastoidectomy reconstruction after surgery. The cavity seen in Figure 7 has been eliminated by reconstruction of the canal wall and the tympanic membrane. Normal epithelial migration has been re-established. The procedure has provided permanent rehabilitation of distressing cavity symptoms.

CHAPTER 9:
TRAUMATIC CONDITIONS OF THE EAR

1. PINNA TRAUMA

(a) Lacerations

Injury to the pinna, as with facial trauma, involves a cosmetically sensitive site. Precise closure, with particular attention to cartilage fragment approximation, is required to avoid troublesome disfiguration. These repairs are preferably undertaken in specialist hands.

(b) Haematoma Auris

Haematoma of the pinna, a classic footballer's or boxer's injury, comprises a collection of blood between the elastic cartilage and the overlying perichondrium. The loss of vascular supply to the cartilage results in a danger of avascular necrosis of the cartilage and therefore a risk of collapse and shrivelling of the normal ear contours with concurrent thickening and fibrosis of the haematoma site, producing the classic "cauliflower ear". To abort this chain of events, evacuation of the haematoma is required to allow re-approximation of the cartilage and its vascular supply. Evacuate by sterile aspiration if the blood collection is fluctuant, or by incision and removal of a solid clot, also under sterile conditions, to avoid perichondritis. In both cases pressure dressings for 2-3 days are advised to prevent re-accumulation. Careful application of pads medial and lateral to the pinna avoids pressure points.

2. TRAUMA TO THE EXTERNAL CANAL

External canal lacerations and abrasions are a common cause of referral to the specialist otologist. Frequent causes are penetrating wounds, self-trauma, insects and their removal, and, regrettably, doctors. The injury is often minor, but blood clots and wax in the external meatus frequently obscure details of the tympanic membrane, rendering interpretation of the situation difficult for the primary care physician.

Clean the external canal by suction, preferably under the operating microscope. This allows evaluation of the tympanic membrane and ossicular chain plus removal of a potential source of infection. If the tympanic membrane is intact, topical antibiotic cream will minimise infections and maximise the chances of rapid healing. Do not initiate ear drop therapy before the state of the tympanic membrane is known. Refer cases where middle ear damage is suspected.

3. TYMPANIC MEMBRANE TRAUMA

The causes of tympanic membrane injuries are similar to those of external meatal trauma, plus those injuries induced by slapping, blast, hot particles and syringing. The presentation is also similar, although a proportion of neglected cases will present later with active otorrhoea due to secondary middle ear infection. Perforations of the tympanic membrane due to burns, eg. welding accidents, are of particular concern, as these tend to a higher incidence of permanent perforations.

On examination, the perforation type depends on the injury. A direct penetration injury tends to cause a bloody gouging perforation, whereas those due to a slap or blast tend towards the appearance of a dry hole, tear or wedge shape defect. Lesions secondary to syringing are frequently delayed in presentation and take on the appearance of the rounded and discharging defect more commonly found in chronic otitis media. Syringing is a frequent cause of tympanic membrane perforation due to a number of factors:

(a) Uncertainty regarding the state of the tympanic membrane, eg. atrophy

(b) A water stream directed at the tympanic membrane rather than the canal wall

(c) Movement of the patient

(d) Movement of the syringing hands

4. OSSICULAR CHAIN TRAUMA

(a) Aetiology

(i) Penetrating injuries (including surgery)

(ii) Blast

(iii) Temporal bone fractures

A drum perforation frequently accompanies this pathology. In fractures of the temporal bone a haemotympanum may be present, possibly with a bloody or CSF otorrhoea. After the drum heals, a conductive deafness persists (Weber to the affected ear, Rinne negative on that side: see Chapter 1) and ossicular aberrations may be seen. Attic fixation, dislocated incus, and stapes and superstructure fractures are common. Audiometry confirms the presence of a conductive loss and tympanometry may show increased compliance on that side. Radiology may show a temporal bone fracture.

(b) Management

If a substantial conductive loss is present, a tympanotomy and ossicular chain reconstruction are undertaken. Good results are usual because the ear is otherwise healthy.

5. EAR TRAUMA DUE TO TEMPORAL BONE FRACTURES

The majority of temporal bone fractures fall into two categories: (Fig. 52)

(a) Longitudinal

(b) Transverse

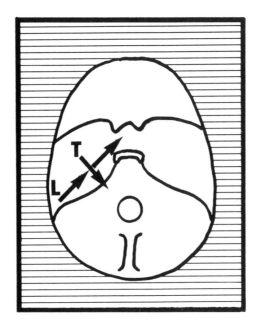

Figure 52.   Fractures of the temporal bone. L: longitudinal; T: transverse.

(a) Longitudinal

(i) Pathology

The fracture line descends across the squamous temporal, sometimes as a barely discernible hairline shadow on plain films. The fracture then passes anteromedially through the roof of the external canal and possibly the attic of the middle ear, but skirting lateral to the hard bony mass of the otic capsule. The facial nerve may be compromised in its middle ear or mastoid course.

(ii) Presentation

The history is of a blow to the side of the head. Bloody or CSF otorrhoea may be present, with deafness on the affected side. Inspection of the canal may be obscured by CSF or blood. Gentle suction toilet permits visualisation of the canal and drum. The fracture may present as a tear in the external meatus, sparing the drum. Alternatively, a haemotympanum or TM rupture may be observed. A conductive loss on tuning fork testing may be shown, but the contralateral ear must be masked to avoid a false Rinne due to sensorineural damage.

(iii) Management is to observe in the early phase, providing high dose, broadspectrum antibiotic cover if a CSF leak is present. If a secondary otitis media presents, this is treated intensively as for acute otitis media (Chapeter 8). Resolution of the acute phase will then permit re-assessment of the hearing in "cold" conditions followed by the appropriate tympanoplasty if indicated.

(b) Transverse

Clinically these amount to approximately 20% of temporal bone fractures, and are due to severe anteroposterior blows. Probably many visit the morgue rather than the clinician.

(i) Pathology

The fracture line passes from the posterior fossa in the region of the internal auditory meatus, laterally through the otic capsule, rending and destroying the labyrinth. Fixed within its bony canal, the facial nerve may fall victim to the shearing effect of the fracture itself.

(ii) Presentation

The general condition of the patient is usually critical due to the severity of the head injury. Upon recovery of consciousness, gross vertigo and total sensorineural deafness are detected, the former gradually stabilising over weeks or months, depending on the concurrent central nervous system state. Facial palsy may go unnoticed until recovery of consciousness.

(iii) Investigation

Radiology to identify the fracture site incorporates plain films, tomography and computerised tomography, and may be valuable in cases of persistent CSF leak or VII palsy. Audiometry in its various forms (pure tone, tympanometry, evoked response testing) is used to assess the extent and nature of the hearing loss. If vertigo persists, electronystagmography is used to assess the site and extent of the loss of vestibular function. Progressive function conduction tests of the VII nerve help guide the surgeon in cases of severe VII palsy. (See "Facial Palsy").

6. BAROTRAUMA IN THE MIDDLE EAR

(a) Aetiology

This condition occurs during episodes of increasing atmospheric pressure. In these conditions, such as diving or descent in an aircraft, aeration of the middle ear may become impeded due to blockage of the eustachian tube. This generally occurs when the external pressure exceeds middle ear pressure by more than 90mm of mercury. Prior pathology, such as upper respiratory tract infections may, however, hinder the eustachian tubal function in conditions of lesser pressure gradients. In cases of severe pressure gradients, tympanic membrane rupture or inner ear complications may result.

(b) Presentation

The patient generally gives a history of recent barotraumatic conditions such as flying or diving. A stuffy or watery feeling is felt in the ear shortly thereafter, together with partial deafness and possibly otalgia. On examination, serous fluid, yellow in colour, possibly together with bubbles in fluid levels, is noted behind the drum. Middle ear haemorrhages or rupture of the tympanic membrane are also occasionally noted.

(c) Management

Prevention of these conditions is best achieved by avoiding the predisposing circumstances whilst an upper respiratory tract infection is present. For those cases who usually have slight eustachian dysfunction in these situations, pseudephedrine and antihistamines given well before the event may be beneficial, together with topical nasal decongestants, swallowing and rapid Valsalva manoeuvres. In established cases, management is either medical or surgical depending on the wishes of the patient. Medical management is similar to the prevention techniques above and will often help settle the situation in a few days. If more urgent relief is desired, a myringotomy or grommet insertion under topical anaesthesia is easily accomplished and gives immediate relief. Temporary mini-grommet insertion before an aircraft flight is a common requirement in susceptible cases.

7. INNER EAR TRAUMA

7.1 AETIOLOGY

7.1.1 BLAST

7.1.2 BAROTRAUMA

7.1.3 HEAD INJURY

7.1.4 PERILYMPH FISTULA

7.1.5 SURGERY RELATED

7.1.1 BLAST

Inner ear damage secondary to exposure to blast at short range is a frequent cause of sensorineural deafness and tinnitus. The ear affected is generally that closest to the blast. The sensorineural deafness is variable in extent but usually involves the high frequency range. The effect on an individual is idiosyncratic and varies from total deafness to barely noticeable high frequency losses. Deafness is frequently temporary, although severe losses rarely recover to normal.

7.1.2 BAROTRAUMA

The inner ear may be damaged by two mechanisms in these situations:

(a) Round window rupture, secondary to severe external pressure changes;

(b) The "bends", secondary to nitrogen bubbles within the bony confines of the otic capsule. The effects of this are relieved by recompression, usually at 3 atmospheres pressure, although permanent sequelae may remain in severe cases.

7.1.3 SENSORINEURAL DEAFNESS DUE TO HEAD INJURY

Sensorineural deafness is a common result of severe head injury. The extent of the loss varies from mild high frequency losses to complete deafness. Severe trauma, involving skull fractures, are more likely to produce these losses. In nonfracture cases the losses tend to be idiosyncratic, as with noise trauma, and recovery in the high frequency losses may occur. If a perilymph fistula is present, vertigo and deafness may be more marked. Exploration is indicated in these cases to detect and seal the fistula.

7.1.4 PERILYMPH FISTULA

Leakage of the perilymph from either the oval or round window occurs due to several causes:

(a) Implosion situations:

(i) Barotrauma

(ii) Blast

(iii) Acoustic trauma

(iv) Post-traumatic

(b) Explosive situations:

   (i) Spontaneous

   (ii) Raised intracranial pressure due to exertion.

PRESENTATION

A history of exposure to an initiating factor will often be present, although in the spontaneous group no known cause can be found. The patient's hearing will usually be severely affected, possibly with a fluctuating sensorineural loss. Vertigo is variable but often severe, and will vary in nature from severe rotatory vertigo to a sensation of unsteadiness. Associated signs due to the initiating factor may also be present, such as fluid in the middle ear or evidence of blast injury to the tympanic membrane. A fistula sign (vertigo and nystagmus) may be elicited utilising a pneumatic speculum to vary external meatal pressure.

MANAGEMENT

Absolute bed rest is indicated, with the head up and the affected ear upwards. The patient is forbidden to undertake manoeuvres which will increase intracranial pressure, and serial audiometry is performed to detect any evidence of fluctuant hearing loss. If a continuing fistula is strongly suspected despite these measures, the ear is explored in an endeavour to seal the leak of perilymph. If such surgery is successful, relief of the vertigo may be obtained and hearing losses may improve.

7.1.5 SURGERY RELATED AETIOLOGY

(a) Post-stapedectomy. A small minority of patients suffer sensorineural deafness after this surgery, varying from minor losses to "dead ears". The cause is often uncertain.

(b) Penetration of the bony labyrinth during cholesteatoma or chronic middle ear surgery.

(c) Concussion trauma secondary to a rotating drill touching the ossicular chain.

(d) Manipulation of diseased ossicles.

(e) Deliberate destruction, eg. labyrinthectomy for Meniere's disease.

Mild high frequency sensorineural losses subsequent to routine middle ear surgery are occasionally observed. The precise cause of this is uncertain, but presumably is secondary to manipulation of the tympanic membrane and ossicular chain during the surgery.

8. RADIATION TRAUMA

Because of its relationship to such structures as the parotid and the postnasal space, the ear may be included in an irradiated field. Regrettably, several severe side effects may result:

(a) Persistent otitis externa:
The delicate external canal skin poorly withstands infection superimposed on radiation damage. Abolishing such infections generally requires meticulous serial suction toilet and antibiotic wick insertions. Gentamicin is of great advantage in these cases.

(b) Sequestration:
Breakdown of the external canal skin may result in a large sequestrum formation. Intractable pain may necessitate complicated excision and vital flap rotation techniques.

(c) Conductive deafness:
Middle ear effusions and fibrosis may result from irradiation of the eustachian tube and the middle ear mucosa. These changes may compromise ossicular vibration, resulting in conductive losses up to 60db in extent.

(d) Sensorineural deafness:
Progressive ipsilateral losses are well documented and may be severe. These losses usually occur after cessation of therapy and are irreversible.

CHAPTER 10:
CONDITIONS OF THE INNER EAR: CLINICAL PRESENTATIONS

1. VERTIGO

2. SENSORINEURAL DEAFNESS

3. THE DEAF CHILD

INTRODUCTION

The inner ear is an organ of both hearing and balance. Disease therefore results in damage to these functions, causing the cardinal symptoms of inner ear disease: tinnitus, deafness (hearing defects), and vertigo (aberrations of balance). Because of the proximity of the cochlea and vestibule, disease often results in combinations of the above symptoms, although purely cochlear or vestibular aberrations are not uncommon. Thorough interrogation will give a clear indication of the diagnosis in many cases.

1. VERTIGO

Vertigo literally means "to go around" but is commonly interchanged with "dizziness" or "giddiness". Otologists prefer to confine the use of "vertigo" to unsteadiness which incorporates a sensation of rotation or spinning as this sensation is frequently associated with an inner ear condition and is thus of particular interest to the ear surgeon. Unsteadiness in general is a common complaint in the primary care situation and results from a wide spectrum of illnesses. Its investigation is essentially that of checking a biological computer system for a fault. As some of the causative lesions are urgent in nature or potentially lethal in the long term, early referral of cases of unsteadiness is advocated. Whether to refer to a neurologist or a neuro-otologist depends on the presentation. In general, patients with sensations of true vertigo (rotation or spinning) or with associated ear symptoms (deafness or tinnitus in particular) should be referred to the otologist, whereas non-rotatory cases may indicate the need for a neurological opinion.

1.1 HISTORY

As unsteadiness can be due to a large number of causes, and as many cases are of minor significance, history-taking attempts to define precisely the symptom, its course and related events.

The patient should be questioned thoroughly regarding the presenting complaint:

(a) **Onset:**
When the problem first occurred and particularly if any explanatory incident occurred at the time or just before.

(b) **Duration**
of the history of the illness, plus the length of each attack.

(c) **Frequency**
of episodes: Note if this is worsening, lessening or stable.

(d) **Severity:**
Particularly if nauseating or incapacitating.

(e) **Nature:**
This is most important. Question for rotation - this may indicate an ear disease origin. Blackouts or syncope indicate a central nervous system origin.

(f) **Location:**
Other ear symptoms may suggest an otological origin. Headaches suggest a CNS site. Other CNS signs may help localise a lesion within the CNS.

(g) **Aggravating or relieving factors:**
Note particularly changes in posture, neck positions or stress. Relief with labyrinthine sedatives such as prochlorperazine may suggest an otological problem.

(h) **Associated factors:**
Ear or central nervous system disease or symptoms help locate the lesion. Note any medication, particularly anti-hypertensive agents which may be contributory.

(i) Otological
Check for otalgia, otorrhoea, tinnitus or deafness.

(ii) Central Nervous System:
Enquire regarding general CNS symptoms (headache, clumsiness, fits, blackouts) or localising symptoms (visual disturbances, weakness, numbness).

Interrogate with regards general health, particularly hypertension, diabetes or psychological illnesses.

1.2 EXAMINATION

(a) Otological

(i) Membrane inspection, tuning fork testing and clinical hearing tests are used to identify ear abnormalities. Test particularly for sensorineural deafness.

(ii) Routine nose and throat examination follows.

(b) CNS

A full clinical examination is performed. Emphasis is placed on cerebellar testing, and testing of V, VII, IX, X and XI (because of their relation to the IAM). Care is taken to check for the effects of tertiary syphilis.

(c) Other

(i) Cervical spine - for cervical spondylosis.

(ii) Endocrine system (thyroid, adrenals).

(iii) Cardiovascular system.

(iv) Evidence of rheumatoid or other autoimmune disease.

1.3 DIFFERENTIAL DIAGNOSIS OF VERTIGO

1.3.1 DISORDERS OF THE LABYRINTH

(a) Middle ear abnormalities

(i) Serous otitis

(ii) Gross destruction by cholesteatoma

(b) Infection

(i) Labyrinthitis - viral

- suppurative

- syphilitic

(c) Trauma

(i) Benign positional vertigo

(ii) Head injury

(iii) Post-stapedectomy

(d) Ototoxics

Aminoglycocides (streptomycin, gentamicin)

(e) Ischaemia

(f) Meniere's Disease

1.3.2 DISORDERS OF THE EIGHTH NERVE AND CENTRAL NERVOUS SYSTEM CONNECTIONS

(a) Vestibular neuronitis

(b) Acoustic neuroma (or other cerebellopontine angle lesions)

(c) Ischaemia:

(i) Vertebro-basilar insufficiency

(ii) Posterior inferior cerebellar artery ischaemia

(d) Disseminated sclerosis

(e) CNS tumours

(f) Autoimmune disease

(g) Syphilis

(h) Migraine

(i) Epilepsy

(j) AIDS

1.3.3 OTHERS

(a) Nuchal vertigo

(b) Psychogenic

(c) Idiopathic group

1.4 INVESTIGATION

(a) Pure Tone Audiometry

This graph of hearing is often of considerable value. Certain illnesses produce a characteristic, sometimes diagnostic pattern such as the low frequency fluctuating sensorineural loss of Meniere's Disease. Noise trauma patterns are often associated with unsteadiness. If normal pure tone audiometry results are obtained, dangerous ear conditions are less likely.

(b) Reflex Testing

The stapedius and tensor tympani reflexes decay in cases of acoustic neuroma. This is readily detected by impedance audiometry.

(c) Evoked Response Audiometry (Electrocochleography, Auditory Brainstem Responses)

Using an averaging computer to eliminate random brain activity waves, the responses of the ear and its central connections are studied to detect defects or distortions of the response to sound "clicks". The tests help to localise the site of lesion.

(d) Speech Discrimination Audiometry

Speech discrimination is often poor in cases of retro-cochlear (VIII nerve) disease.

(e) Electronystagmography

Cases of vertigo commonly present with nystagmus which is present constantly or may be provoked. The nature and severity of nystagmus is recorded and tests are used to determine if the nystagmus can be initiated or worsened by cervical spine movements or postural changes. Direction changing nystagmus, provoked by looking first right, then left, may indicate a CNS lesion. Caloric tests show the presence or absence of a vestibular palsy and if positive, are strongly suggestive of ear disease in the affected side.

(f) *Radiology*

In a case of vertigo, it is essential to ascertain as clearly as possible whether or not an IAM lesion is present. Failure to do so may result in an acoustic neuroma being missed. CT and MRI scans are used. The latter is optimal for small soft tissue lesions although claustrophobia is an occasional problem and may dictate sedation.

(g) *Pathology*

(i) Serological tests are performed to exclude syphilis (VDRL, TPHA) and HIV.

(ii) Hormonal assays to exclude thyroid or adrenal abnormalities.

(iii) Full blood count, ESR.

(iv) Autoimmune screen to exclude polyarteritis, temporal arteritis.

(v) CSF studies if indicated on clinical grounds.

(h) *Electroencephalography*

EEG recordings are made to exclude central nervous system diseases if the CNS is considered to be the site of origin of the vertigo (eg. epilepsy).

2. SENSORINEURAL DEAFNESS

Sensorineural, nerve or perceptive deafness results from damage to the cochlea or its central connections. The losses are unilateral or bilateral and either stable, fluctuant or deteriorating. Stable losses often result from "one off" causes, (eg. trauma, vascular occlusion) and are not urgent in nature. Fluctuant or deteriorating cases, however, are otological emergencies requiring prompt management to minimise further losses which are often irreversible.

2.1 HISTORY

Examining the features of sensorineural deafness requires an interrogative process similar to that used for vertigo.

2.2. PRESENTING SYMPTOMS

(a) The onset and duration or the loss are established.

(b) *Severity.*

Ascertain the extent of the loss and particularly if it is stable or fluctuant.

(c) *Nature.*

Inability to hear certain sounds may indicate the type of the loss. In high frequency losses, sounds such as the telephone bell or some consonants may not be heard.

(d) *Location.*

Establish whether the loss is unilateral or bilateral. Diseases causing bilateral losses (eg. noise, ototoxics)

are less likely to cause a unilateral loss as found in acoustic neuroma.

(e) *Aggravating or relieving factors.*

The patient may have noticed worsening influences (eg. noise) or relieving factors (eg. use of steroids in late syphilis).

(f) *Associated symptoms*

due to ear, CNS or other disease may give a lead to the correct diagnosis.

2.3 EXAMINATION

As in cases of vertigo a thorough ear and CNS examination is performed.

2.4 INVESTIGATION

The investigation of sensorineural deafness is similar to the methods used to probe cases of vertigo, but tests of balance are not performed routinely if there is no history of unsteadiness. The extent of the audiological and radiological assessment is indicated by the history and initial audiological findings, eg. bilateral high frequency symmetrical losses in an eighty-year-old (age losses) warrant only pure tone audiometry, in contrast to a unilateral deteriorating loss in a sixty-year-old, which might herald an acoustic neuroma. Such a case would be fully investigated.

2.5 DIFFERENTIAL DIAGNOSIS

2.5.1 LABYRINTHINE DISEASE

(a) *Presbyacusis*

(b) *Infection:*
(i) bacterial

(ii) viral

(c) *Ototoxics*

(d) *Trauma*

(e) *Vascular disease*

(f) *Meniere's disease*

(g) *Autoimmune diseases.*

2.5.2 ACOUSTIC NERVE

(a) *Trauma*

(b) *Meningitis*

(c) *Tumours*

(d) *Disseminated sclerosis*

2.5.3 CNS DISEASE

2.5.4 NON-ORGANIC

3. THE DEAF CHILD

Deafness in an infant or child represents a major developmental problem, capable of severely retarding the child's learning ability. The problem is not readily apparent and is easily missed.

3.1 AETIOLOGY

The deafness can be either conductive or sensorineural. The conductive types are dealt with in full in the relevant chapters elsewhere in this book. Sensorineural deafness in the child is either congenital or acquired. Severe losses in young children are of considerable concern, as they not infrequently deteriorate markedly, without apparent cause.

3.1.1 PRENATAL CAUSES

(a) Genetic Origin

The deafness may be part of a wider pathological picture (eg. Pendreds Syndrome, Klippel Feil Syndrome), or it may be confined to the inner ear alone, (eg. Scheibe deformities).

(b) Acquired

A large range of intrauterine or perinatal diseases can cause deafness. Common causes are:

(i) Infection (rubella, chicken pox)

(ii) Ototoxics

(iii) Metabolic factors:
* diabetes
* nephritis
* toxaemia

3.1.2 NATAL & PERINATAL CAUSES

(a) Birth trauma

(b) Anoxia

(c) Infections

(d) Kernicterus

(e) Prematurity

(f) Others (metabolic, ototoxics, etc.)

3.1.3 POSTNATAL CAUSES

(a) Congenital Defects
(i) Familial sensorineural deafness

(ii) Alports Syndrome

(b) Acquired Sensorineural Deafness
(i) Infections: measles, mumps, meningitis

(ii) Trauma

(iii) Ototoxics

(iv) Anoxia

3.2 PRESENTATION

The clinical picture depends on the age of the child. Many reach 1-2 years of age before detection. Prior to assessment, the external auditory meati are cleaned and the drums inspected to eliminate the possibility of a middle or external ear disease. If both are clear, conductive deafness is possible but unlikely.

3.2.1 INFANTS

The history is one of suspicion on the part of the mother or the child's attendants. Failure to respond to sounds by blinking and movement may be noted. In neonates, the Moro reflex may be absent upon stimulation with louder sounds.

3.2.2 OLDER CHILDREN

When children begin to sit up (7-9 months), they also begin to acquire the ability to turn towards sounds. Sounds at various pitches (rattles, whistles) may be used to gain a crude assessment of frequency loss (eg. as most sensorineural losses will incorporate a high frequency loss, a high frequency sound may be missed.)

In older children, assessment of the child's speech ability may also be helpful. Primitive speech ("da", "ha", "ba", etc) appears around 28 weeks and proceeds to double syllables ("ta-ta", "da-da") at about 32 weeks. A few single words with meaning ("toy", "mum") may be spoken at one year. Word linkage and sentence development progresses in the 18- 24 months period, with pronouns ("I", "me", "you") being in use at two years. By three years, a good basic understanding and use of language should have been mastered and the child should understand quiet speech at one metre. If deafness in a child is missed or left untreated, a spectrum of problems will result. The deaf child has a special handicap which:

(i) is invisible;

(ii) retards progress;

(iii) may produce behaviour aberrations.

3.3 CHARACTERISTICS OF THE DEAF CHILD

(a) Mild   misses conversation (lip reads)
noted at school
noted by mother
inattentive, vague, daydreams

(b) Medium   loud TV
misbehaves, hyperactive
pronounced school problems

(c) Severe   speech failure, obvious hearing defect

3.4 RESULTS OF CHILDHOOD DEAFNESS

(a) Mild-moderate

punishment for "inattentiveness"
poor school progress
slight speech problems

(b) Severe

gross speech retardation
personality problems
ostracised by fellows
teased - "deafy" etc.

If deafness is suspected on clinical examination, investigate the child thoroughly.

3.5 HISTORY AND EXAMINATION OF THE DEAF CHILD

Clinically one aims to establish:

(a) if deafness is present, and if so

(b) which type, and

(c) what cause

3.5.1 HISTORY

(a) Deafness. Establish site, duration, onset, severity, nature (e.g. high frequency), aggravating/relieving factors.

(b) Other ear symptoms (pain, discharge, tinnitus, vertigo). Question these exhaustively along the usual lines.

(c) Associated symptoms.

3.5.2 EXAMINATION

(a) Inspect the ears. (These must be clean). A thorough knowledge of the variations of the normal drum, plus the pathological states, is essential. Inspect all the drum, including the pars flaccida.

(b) Speech testing. Mask one ear by rustling paper. Test the hearing vocally as per Chapter I. Tuning fork testing is not usually of help in children.

(c) Other areas. Check upper respiratory tract and CNS for cause of deafness.

3.5.3 AUDIOLOGY

An increased range of test procedures has lowered the age for hearing measurement down to neonates.

(a) Behavioural Observation Audiometry

In young infants, subtle changes to a variety of sound field auditory stimuli provide an indication of hearing across the frequency range.

(b) Condition Orientation Response (COR)

The older infant produces a turning response to sound and this can be visually reinforced. Sound field thresholds can be obtained for warble tones and individual ears and bone conduction measures can also be obtained if co-operation is sufficient.

(c) Pure Tone Audiometry

If the child is co-operative, using play techniques, an adult type audiogram can be obtained by about 3 years. The reliability of the measures will improve with developmental age.

(d) Acoustic Immittance Measures

Middle ear measures (tympanometry) are widely used to exclude eustachian tube dysfunction, which is a common cause of childhood deafness.

(e) Acoustic Reflex Measures

Acoustic reflex measures form part of the clinical acoustic immittance procedure and provide an indication of cochlear hearing levels, particularly by comparison of broad band (white noise) and pure tone acoustic reflex sensation levels.

(f) Auditory Brainstem Response (ABR)

The ABR waveform is a reliable indication of hearing levels in the higher frequencies. Variations using tone bursts and bone conduction stimuli provide additional information about the audiogram. Sedation or G.A. could be required to avoid overshadowing the response by muscle activity.

(g) Oto-acoustic Emissions

The "cochlear echo", which can be recorded from the ear canal with a probe microphone following tonal stimulation and computer analysis is increasingly important as an objective measure of hearing.

3.6 MANAGEMENT OF THE DEAF CHILD

(a) Treatment of causative condition

is undertaken, if possible, to minimise further loss.

(b) Hearing Aids.

In many cases of hearing loss of lesser extent, binaural hearing aids may help children obtain normal schooling. Severe cases with speech discrimination problems will require further help despite the aids.

(c) Speech Therapy

Professional tuition is required in severe cases to develop speech. Therapy seeks to teach the child to first listen, then to talk. Speech can be developed in even severely deaf children, using hearing aids. The profoundly deaf child may require a cochlear implant to develop full vocal ability. Great advances are now possible using these devices.

(d) Alternative Communication.

Where speech development is not practicable, lipreading

and sign language provide alternative communication modes. These have been widely used in the past but are now being replaced in many cases by the technology of cochlear implants.

(e) Cochlear Implants.

Cochlear implants are used in profound losses which cannot benefit adequately from the use of hearing aids. The "bionic ear" incorporates a 22 electrode array inserted into the cochleca spiral. The array is attached to an implanted receiver (an induction coil). (Figs. 53, 54)

mitter) receives and processes sounds. The processor then stimulates the implanted receiver by means of an external induction coil. The sound received is described by adult implantees as being crude but semi-recognisable ("Donald Duck" or "a radio station slightly out of tune"). Implants have proven a major advance in the management of both adult and paediatric profound sensorineural deafness. If implanted early, suitable children may achieve near-normal speech and hearing, although only after intensive habilitation (speech training).

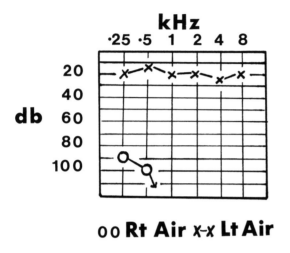

Figure 53. Severe sensorineural deafness in the right ear. If bilateral this patient would be extremely limited in auditory communication and would probably require a cochlear implant.

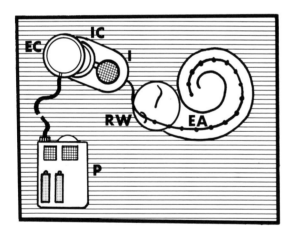

Figure 54. Plan of the cochlear implant. The external micro-processor (P) receives sounds, encodes these into electrical impulses and stimulates the implanted prosthesis via the external electromagnetic coil (EC). The implanted prosthesis receives the impulses via the internal induction coil (IC). The impulses are processed in the implanted electronics and the cochlea is then stimulated via twenty-two electrodes implanted into the cochlear spiral on the electrode array (EA). RW: round window.

An external receiver (microphone, transducer and trans-

CHAPTER 11:
CONDITIONS OF THE INNER EAR: CLINICAL CONDITIONS

The inner ear may exhibit a wide range of clinical conditions.

1. FAMILIAL DEAFNESS

Progressive or stable sensorineural losses with an attendant family history of similar problems are a common clinical entity. A range of genetic patterns is involved. The deafness may be a mid-frequency U-shaped loss (Fig. 55) which may go unnoticed for many years. Other patients present with progressive high frequency sensorineural losses which may progress to total bilateral deafness. Little preventative treatment is available. Hearing aids are required or possibly cochlear implantation in severe cases.

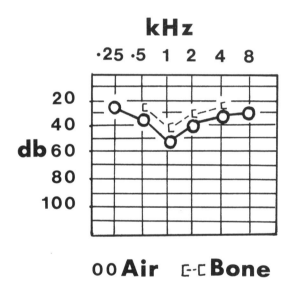

kHz
·25 ·5 1 2 4 8

oo **Air**   ᴇ-ᴄ **Bone**

Figure 55. Congenital deafness. A mid-frequency U-shaped loss is typical of a genetically determined loss.

2. PRESBYACUSIS

Deafness is an inevitable consequence of age. Its onset varies from the early fifth decade onwards, although many people retain good hearing until late in life. The progressive loss of hearing is accompanied by a more subtle loss of vestibular function, although the latter undergoes compensation and is therefore less of a problem.

2.1 AETIOLOGY AND PATHOLOGY

The loss of hearing is due to gradual degeneration of the cochlea, particularly the organ of Corti. There are few strongly recognised aetiological factors, although urban man appears to be more prone to the process, possibly as a result of chronic exposure to high noise levels.

2.2 PRESENTATION

The aged patient will present with several major symptoms. Pain and otorrhoea are not a feature of presbyacusis.

(a) Deafness

The loss of hearing is classically high frequency in distribution. The patient often notices his inability to hear a telephone bell at a distance. Speech discrimination is reduced due to the loss of the consonants, particularly those with a hissing quality.

(b) Tinnitus

Tinnitus is frequently present and may be the presenting complaint. This is generally high pitched or buzzing in nature, often unilateral.

(c) Unsteadiness

Unsteadiness due to vestibular dysfunction is frequently present although this may be intermittent as the patient compensates for the loss of this function.

On examination, the ears appear normal, apart from the clinical deafness. Tuning fork testing usually fails to show a unilateral problem as the loss is generally symmetrical.

2.3 INVESTIGATION

Audiometry is frequently diagnostic in these cases, showing a symmetrical, sloping high frequency sensorineural deafness. (Fig. 56)

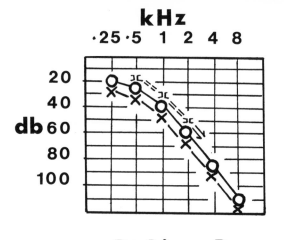

oo Rt Air ⊏-⊏ **Bone**
xx Lt Air ⊐-⊐ **Bone**

Figure 56.   Presbyacusis. A symmetrical bilateral high frequency sensorineural loss is seen in an elderly patient. In such cases the losses are pathognomonic of presbyacusis.

2.4 MANAGEMENT

Upon diagnosis of the condition, the patient should be reassured that the problem is a normal consequence of age. Most such patients have contemporaries with similar problems, and many are reassured that there is nothing worse present. In those patients in whom the hearing is becoming difficult, lipreading during conversation is helpful. This is also a considerable advantage if hearing aids are used. The latter generally become helpful when the speech frequencies (250-2000 cycles per second) are reduced approximately 30-35 decibels. If an aid is to be supplied, the patient should be warned this will be of most advantage in quiet situations and that noisy conditions will render the aid of little help. Regrettably many cases, due to uneven loss of hearing, obtain little help from an aid due to impairment of their speech discrimination ability. In addition, many such cases suffer recruitment. This is a distortion of speech due to enhanced perception of the sound received. Recruitment and speech discrimination loss are major problems in many elderly people. In these cases, lipreading is even more important. Current aid technology tailors the amplification pattern of the aid to the individual with significant improvement in sound quality.

3.   NOISE TRAUMA

3.1   INTRODUCTION

Chronic exposure to noise of higher than 70 decibels intensity results in gradual loss of hearing. This condition, referred to as "boilermaker's ear" etc, is a growing area of awareness in workers' compensation cases.

3.2   PATHOLOGY

High noise levels sustained for more than three minutes at a time cause, with time, permanent damage to the organ of Corti including destruction of the hair cells. The cells of the basal turn of the cochlea, particularly opposite the oval window, are those most affected. (Fig. 57)

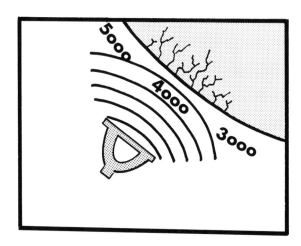

Figure 57.   Concussive effects of noise. The hair cells opposite the stapes suffers the most damage.

The cells opposite the window are those responsible for detection of the 4000 cycles per second range. Due to their proximity to the entrance of the noise, these are most prone to damage. Destruction in this area is noted clinically by maximal losses at 4000 cycles per second. With time, further progressive damage occurs in the adjacent areas of the cochlea. This is accompanied by a progressive loss of function in the associated higher tones, usually in the 2000-8000 cycles per second range. (Fig. 58)

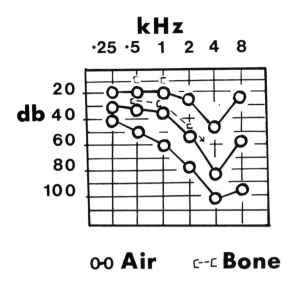

kHz

·25 ·5 1 2 4 8

db 20 40 60 80 100

o–o **Air**   c–c **Bone**

Figure 58.   Pure tone audiometry in noise trauma. The losses begin as an isolated loss of four thousand cycles per second then gradually progress with damage to the adjacent frequencies.

3.3 PRESENTATION

(a) History

The primary presentation is that of deafness. The patient may have noticed that this is more in the high pitched range, similar to the presbyacusic patient. The problems are due to the loss of the high frequencies. In old patients, it may be clinically impossible to discern between noise deafness and presbyacusis due to the similarity of loss in both conditions. The patient may give a firm history of exposure to noise in industry, sport (eg. shooting), or as a result of war service. Tinnitus may be a major problem and is due to cochlear damage with resultant malfunction of the sensory cells. "Electronic" sounds such as whistling, buzzing or ringing are typical. Pain and discharge are absent, and although not common, balance problems, usually transient unsteadiness, may be part of the clinical picture.

(b) Signs

Sensorineural deafness is present and usually bilateral, although often unequal. Worse loss in the left ear may follow rifle shooting. This ear, being closer to the muzzle of the weapon, may be subject to more blast than the right. The tympanic membranes appear normal. The Weber in most cases will be central and the Rinnes bilaterally positive.

3.4 INVESTIGATION

Pure tone audiometry is typical in most cases. A high frequency sensorineural loss, with the characteristic dip at 4000 cycles per second, is diagnostic. In very early cases, the 4000 cps frequency alone may be afflicted, but in more severe cases there is a progressive loss of the frequencies as a whole,

more in the higher frequencies. Diagnosis may be more difficult in more severe cases which may closely resemble presbyacusis. This is a particular problem in the older age group when considering a case for workers' compensation. For such cases, government agencies have issued guidelines of allowances for age. Cases of excessive loss are usually given the benefit of the doubt.

3.5 MANAGEMENT

Once established, sensorineural deafness cannot be corrected. Noise trauma prevention is the major form of management. Fortunately health authorities are aware of the problem and mitigation of industrial noise levels for protection of the worker in such an environment is a well-established art. Protection takes the form of ear muffs and plugs. Of these, the muffs are the more efficient. Silencing machinery or buffering noisy plant may be undertaken. Health inspectors should inspect noisy areas regularly.

If a loss has occurred, treatment is directed to improving the individual's ability to communicate. Hearing aids may help, although the uneven nature of the hearing loss causes technical problems in amplifying sound in these cases. Lipreading, which is often developed by the patient on an involuntary basis, is valuable to the patient especially when used in conjunction with a hearing aid. Other ancillary aids include modifying the tone of the telephone bell to a lower pitch and providing a volume control on the individual's telephone.

4.   OTOTOXICITY

The inner ear is sensitive to a number of chemotherapeutic substances. A range of modern drugs has been implicated. The most important are:

    1. Aminoglycoside antibiotics
    2. Salicylates
    3. Antimalarials
    4. Diuretics
    5. Others

4.1 AMINOGLYCOSIDE ANTIBIOTICS

The ototoxic properties of this group of drugs were initially noted in the early treatment of tuberculosis and in their subsequent use in surgery and nephrology. The members of the group fall into either predominantly cochleotoxic or vestibulotoxic groups.

(a) Cochlear Toxicity

    (i)   Dihydrostreptomycin

    (ii) Kanamycin

    (iii) Neomycin

(b) *Vestibular Toxicity*

    (i) Streptomycin

    (ii) Tobramycin

    (iii) Gentamicin

4.1.1 PATHOLOGY

Progressive hair cell damage occurs, with later further organ of Corti damage. The vestibular damage is localised more in the semicircular canals, with damage to both the cellular structures and the cilia. The precise ototoxic mechanism is uncertain.

4.1.2 PRESENTATION

The ototoxicity of these drugs depends primarily on the predominant site of action of the drug concerned. Tinnitus, then high frequency sensorineural deafness, which may appear some time after cessation of the drug, are the frequent presenting signs. These may progress to complete sensorineural deafness. In the second group, vertigo predominates, but is variable in its extent and nature. Progressive deafness may accompany the vertigo.

4.1.3 INVESTIGATION

Pure tone audiometry shows a bilateral high frequency sensorineural loss. ABR shows a cochlear pattern. ENG may show a bilateral vestibular palsy, worse with the vestibulotoxic group.

4.1.4 MANAGEMENT

Established cases are incurable and prevention is essential. This is a complex task, particularly if renal impairment is present. Parenteral administration of these drugs should be confined to skilled practitioners familiar with their use.

4.2 OTHER DRUGS

Ethacrynic Acid and Frusemide have a history of causing sensorineural loss, sometimes reversible, but worsened by concomitant treatment with aminoglycosides. Phenytoin may cause reversible vestibular disturbances. Practolol may cause a delayed onset sensorineural deafness, sometimes associated with a middle ear effusion.

5. BENIGN POSITIONAL PAROXYSMAL VERTIGO (BPPV)

This condition is characterised by episodes of rotatory vertigo precipitated by a change in position. The episodes are short-lived, lasting up to 10-30 seconds, and are noted to come upon the patient when he takes up a specific position. This positional change may be well recognised by the patient (eg. rolling on to the left side in bed). The victim learns to avoid the critical position where possible.

5.1 AETIOLOGY

The condition is often related to a past history of head injury. Some cases at least are thought to be due to debris in the vestibule coming to rest on the posterior semicircular canal cupola. Otoliths released by utricular degeneration may cause some cases.

5.2 SYMPTOMS AND SIGNS

Apart from the above vertigo, there may be no other findings, or these may be coincidental. ENG may show nystagmus in the trigger position without other changes. CNS signs - Rombergs and cerebellar - must be excluded as brainstem lesions may produce a more violent positional vertigo. The latter does not fatigue and is associated with other evidence of CNS disease including the coarse, variable CNS-type nystagmus and cerebellar signs.

5.3 MANAGEMENT

The other major causes of vertigo are excluded and the patient is then counselled regarding the benign nature of the illness and the need to avoid the movements or position which induce the problem. Drugs are of little help in most cases. Surgical ablation of the posterior semicircular canal has been suggested as curative therapy, but remains under assessment.

6. VESTIBULAR NEURONITIS

This is a condition of probable viral origin characterised by rotatory vertigo without other symptoms. The onset may be associated with an upper respiratory tract infection. The initial episode may last several days, gradually abating with residual balance aberrations lasting up to several weeks or months. A fine horizontal nystagmus to the unaffected side may be present. All tests for vertigo are normal, except for the ENG which shows a unilateral vestibular palsy and possibly a spontaneous nystagmus. Particularly, there is no evidence of hearing loss. The management is supportive (Stemetil or Largactil) until spontaneous relief ensues. A proportion of cases may suffer recurrent episodes, sometimes over several months. The condition is frequently confused with viral labyrinthitis, but the latter is associated with sensorineural deafness. (Fig. 59)

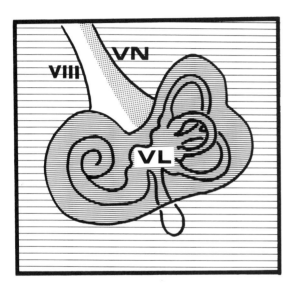

Figure 59. Pathology patterns in vestibular neuronitis and viral labyrinthitis. Vestibular neuronitis affects only the vestibular portion of the eighth nerve. Viral labyrinthitis affects both the cochlear and the lateral semicircular canals. In the latter condition, both deafness and dizziness will be evident. In vestibular neuronitis only dizziness will be present.

7. VIRAL LABYRINTHITIS

Viral labyrinthitis may be due to many agents, including the usual URTI viruses, glandular fever, measles, mumps, chickenpox and herpes zoster (the latter in association with the Ramsay-Hunt syndrome). Variable damage is caused to both the cochlea and the vestibular labyrinth and, because of the variable nature of the pathology, vertigo, tinnitus and sensorineural deafness occur to irregular extents. In cases where vertigo predominates, the condition may be confused with vestibular neuronitis but it is emphasised that pure vertigo without associated deafness in cases of viral labyrinthitis is unusual.

8. ISCHAEMIC INNER EAR DISEASE

8.1 INTRODUCTION

Ischaemia of the inner ear may result from haemodynamic or occlusive origins. Minor inner ear problems of uncertain origin are commonplace and many are probably due to microvascular lesions. Because of the dimensions of the vessels concerned, there are few specific investigations available, but the group should not be used as a diagnostic dumping ground.

8.2 PRESENTATION

Vertebrobasilar insufficiency due to pinching of the vertebral arteries in the neck and base of the skull, particularly on looking up, may produce drop attacks or vertigo in association with brainstem signs. Minor occlusion episodes of the inner ear proper present with tinnitus, sensorineural deafness and vertigo. These symptoms are present to varying degrees and may be exclusively cochlear or vestibular, depending on the vessel concerned. They may thus mimic other disease, eg. trauma or vestibular neuronitis. Diffuse embolic episodes may be associated with focal brainstem or cerebellar signs.

8.3 MANAGEMENT

With significant symptoms, a full audiological/vestibular assessment must be undertaken to exclude major disease, but a large number of cases will result in a diagnosis of sensorineural deafness or vertigo - cause uncertain. Nonetheless, the patient can be reassured in safety and this will be of great relief to those patients who are worried about serious illness. Prochlorperazine or other labyrinthine sedatives may help vertigo. Deafness may require the help of an aid and tinnitus may necessitate distraction techniques (eg. music) or sedation at night.

9. SYPHILITIC INNER EAR DISEASE

Because of its susceptibility to penicillin and the frequent cures obtained in this disease in early cases, syphilis has faded into the background of modern otological practice. It remains a treacherous mimic, however, and may return in greater force in future years. It is noted in two forms:

(a) Acute meningovascular syphilis, found at the secondary stage, and

(b) Late congenital or acquired disease.

(a) *Acute Meningovascular Syphilis*

This manifests at or just after the secondary stage. The patient suffers an endarteritis of the brain and meninges, presenting with headache and fever. This may extend to involve the VIII nerve and labyrinth, causing sensorineural deafness, vertigo and tinnitus. Other cranial nerve palsies and other CNS signs may manifest. There is often a concrete history of an infection contact and the cutaneous lesions of secondary syphilis may be present. The serological tests for syphilis are strongly positive, as are studies on the CSF.

Management is by penicillin, or cephaloridine if the individual is allergic to penicillin, plus steroids to avoid a Herxheimer reaction. Long term follow-up by a specialist venereologist is advised.

(b) Late Syphilis

The presence of inner ear damage due to late syphilis remains an important clinical consideration in the investigation of inner ear disease. It presents perhaps decades after the primary infection, and there may be a history of antitreponemal therapy. The disease may be either congenital or acquired. The patient presents with progressive sensorineural deafness, perhaps fluctuant. Tinnitus and/or vertigo may also be present. The latter may closely resemble true Meniere's disease. Audiology confirms the sensorineural loss, which may include a fluctuant Meniere's-like low frequency sensorineural loss, a pattern rarely found elsewhere. Electronystagmography may show bilateral reduced caloric responses and spontaneous nystagmus. Other clinical manifestations of neurosyphilis may be present and there may be a history of interstitial keratitis. The serology shows positive reactions.

The treatment of choice is combined penicillin and steroid therapy. Benzylpenicillin-G is given, 0.5 megaunits q.i.d, together with probenecid 0.5 grams b.d. to boost serum levels of the penicillin. This is combined with prednisone 10 milligrams t.d.s. for ten days, then 25 milligrams t.d.s. for three weeks. Five milligrams daily is continued on a long term basis. In cases of penicillin allergy, cephaloridine 500 milligrams q.i.d. is given over three weeks. The symptoms can be well controlled by adequate treatment and follow-up, but relapses are common and long term follow-up by a venereologist is essential.

10. MENIERE'S DISEASE (ENDOLYMPHATIC HYDROPS)

True Meniere's disease in its clinical form, outlined below, is an important but not common cause of vertigo and deafness. Regrettably it has become something of a dumping ground for undiagnosed causes of vertigo. This temptation should be resisted by the practitioner, as Meniere's disease as such is a clearly defined entity with unique management, often as a semi-emergency surgical case.

10.1 AETIOLOGY AND PATHOLOGY

Meniere's disease is due to distension of the membranous labyrinth as a result of excessive accumulation of the endolymph contained within (endolympatic hydrops). This distension is secondary to failure of the saccus endolymphaticus to absorb the endolymph normally continually produced within the inner ear. The aetiology of this failure remains uncertain, but may be related to migraine-like vascular spasms. As a result of the ballooning of the membranous labyrinth, widespread cochlear and vestibular damage results and may be associated with rupture of the membranous labyrinth. (Figs. 60, 61)

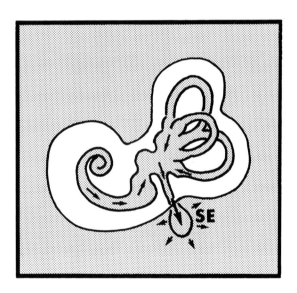

Figure 60.   Normal saccus endolymphaticus function. The saccus resorbs fluid which is continually produced in the membranous labyrinth providing a dynamic replacement of the fluid within the inner ear membranes.

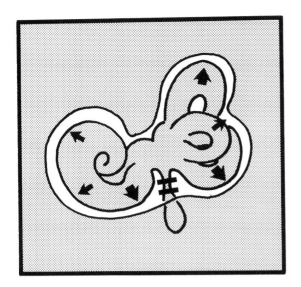

Figure 61. Endolymphatic hydrops. Drainage via the saccus has been impeded and the membranous labyrinth has become distended with endolymph.

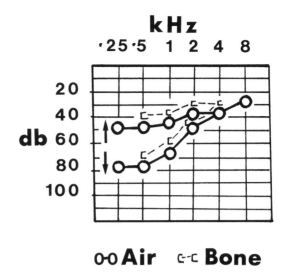

Figure 62. Pure tone audiometry in Meniere's disease. A fluctuant, low frequency sensorineural deafness is present. This is typical of endolymphatic hydrops.

10.2 PRESENTATION

Classically the disease occurs in episodes varying from a few minutes up to several days. Initially the patient notices a feeling of pressure or fullness in the affected ear followed by inner ear-type tinnitus (whistling, ringing etc). Rotatory vertigo, often severe, ensues and may cause nausea and vomiting. Deafness is noticed at the time of the episodes, possibly improving thereafter but progressively worsening with attacks. There is no pain or discharge.

Signs: Acute Phase. During an attack the patient will be dizzy and nauseated. A fine horizontal nystagmus towards the unaffected ear is observed. The Weber is felt in the better ear, and the Rinnes are positive bilaterally. The tympanic membranes are normal on inspection. Between the attacks a sensorineural loss is noted in the affected ear, but there may be no other signs.

10.3 INVESTIGATIONS

(a) Pure Tone Audiometry (PTA)

Meniere's disease produces a characteristic low frequency sensorineural deafness, an audiological pattern rarely found in other conditions. Fluctuation of this loss may be demonstrated and if so is almost diagnostic of Meniere's disease (but beware syphilis). With attacks, the sensorineural loss worsens and if the disease is not arrested it may become total. (Fig. 62)

(b) Evoked Response Audiometry (ECoG, ABR)

This shows loss or distortion of the cochlear microphonic responses produced by sound waves in the inner ear. This indicates damage at the end organ level as found in Meniere's disease at histology.

(c) Electronystagmography (ENG)

This may show a spontaneous nystagmus to the contralateral side and a vestibular palsy on caloric testing of the affected ear.

(d) Radiology

is clear of pathological changes.

(e)

A special test, the Glycerol test, may confirm the diagnosis of Meniere's disease more precisely. A planned amount of Glycerol is given to the patient and as a result of this administration the patient's hearing may improve slightly in cases of true Meniere's disease. The test is helpful in suggesting the surgical management (saccus decompression or drainage) in positive cases.

10.4 MANAGEMENT

Once diagnosed, prompt treatment is indicated to avoid further sensorineural deafness which may be irreversible.

(a) Conservative

(i) Bed rest and sedation

(ii) Prochlorperazine, chlorpromazine, droperidol.

(iii) Betahistine ("Serc") 4mg t.d.s may be effective, but it is emphasised that this is antagonistic with the antihistamines above and should not be administered simultaneously.

(b) Surgery

(i) Saccus endolymphaticus decompression or drainage: In this procedure, the saccus endolymphaticus is exposed via a transmastoid approach and is completely decompressed by removal of the mastoid bony structures lateral to the saccus. A micro-shunt from the sac to the CSF space immediately deep to the sac may also be used. Success rates of 60-70% are claimed in the short term, although long term results are less satisfactory. The mechanism by which this surgery is effective remains ill-understood and controversial.

(ii) In more severe cases of vertigo in which the sensorineural deafness is not severe, the vestibular part of the eighth nerve is sectioned via a posterior or middle fossa approach. This however, has no effect on the outcome of the disease on hearing.

(iii) In severe cases with destruction of the sensorineural reserves of the affected ear, labyrinthectomy via a transcanal or transmastoid approach may effectively eliminate further vertigo. Labyrinthectomy and nerve section are performed with caution on older patients, because of the resultant troublesome unsteadiness in this age group.

(iv) In the case of an only hearing ear, sympathectomy of the cervical chain on the ipsilateral side may be helpful.

11. ACOUSTIC NEUROMA

11.1 INTRODUCTION

Acoustic neuroma is an uncommon benign tumour of the VIII nerve. Because of its lethal potential, it is best diagnosed early to prevent major CNS involvement with its resultant increase in morbidity and mortality.

11.2 PATHOLOGY

The tumour is derived from the Schwann cells of the superior vestibular nerve. Its growth is gradual. Expansion causes erosion of the internal meatus and compression of its contents. Eventual attachment to the brainstem and parasitism of its blood supply occur and this derangement results in inoperability in these advanced cases. (Fig. 63, 64)

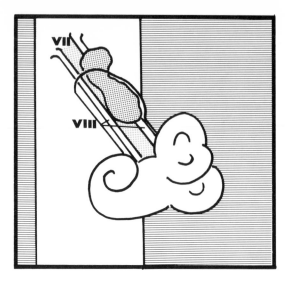

Figure 63.   Acoustic neuroma. The lesion develops on the vestibular nerve in the internal auditory meatus gradually distending the canal and compressing the neural contents.

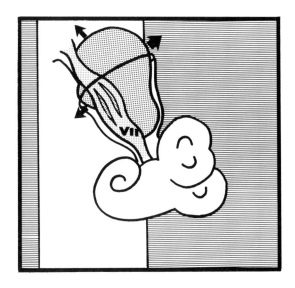

Figure 64.   Advanced acoustic neuroma. The canal has been flared by gradual erosion. The facial nerve is thinned and splayed over the lesion. The tumour may parasitise the blood vessels of the brainstem.

11.3 PRESENTING SYMPTOMS

Sensorineural deafness due to VIII nerve compression is common, but variable in the pattern of the frequencies affected. Sudden severe deafness may result from tumour oedema or haemorrhage. Tinnitus is common. Vertigo due to nerve compression or vascular occlusion varies from transient unsteadiness to a Meniere's disease-like picture, hence the caution required when dealing with all vertigo cases. Pain is uncommon and only vaguely described in some cases as a retroauricular deep ache. Nerve palsies, in association with sensorineural deafness, are strongly indicative of VIII nerve lesions. Compression of the facial nerve in the auditory meatus may produce a progressive paralysis which may however, be reversible with prompt surgery. Larger tumours may cause V nerve impairment, especially the cochlear reflex (V2). Posterior fossa CNS signs indicate a large lesion.

11.4 EXAMINATION

Full otological and CNS examination is undertaken as outlined in the sections on Vertigo and Sensorineural Deafness. (See Chapter 10)

11.5 MANAGEMENT

(a) Investigations

(i) Radiology

Plain films and tomography may demonstrate a flared medial end of the internal auditory meatus. CT scanning identifies lesions down to 1.0cm diameter. MRI scans are the state-of-the-art examination at this time, identifying lesions as small as 2mm.

(ii) Audiology

As pure tone audiometry findings are not specific, sophisticated audiometry tests are required to aid in the diagnosis of small lesions. Enhanced fatigue or "decay" of the acoustic reflexes (tensor tympani and stapedius), measured by impedance audiometry, is noted in these lesions. ABR assessments are an invaluable screening tool. Wave V latency delays are seen on the latter. Positive ABR findings should be followed up with MRI scans. Speech discrimination audiometry may show marked deterioration. Electronystagmography demonstrates a vestibular paresis on the affected side. Tests of facial nerve function may demonstrate a sub-clinical loss of function on the tumour side.

(b) Surgery

is undertaken via one of several routes. If hearing is salvageable, middle fossa or retrosigmoid approaches may be used to preserve this function. If hearing is lost, translabyrinthine, transtentorial or posterior fossa approaches may be used. (Fig. 65) As these lesions may be very slow-growing, surgery may be contra-indicated in very aged or infirm patients.

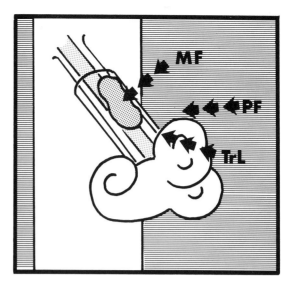

Figure 65.   Surgical approaches to the internal auditory meatus. MF: middle fossa; PF: posterior fossa; TrL: translabyrinthine.

12. GLOMUS TUMOURS

12.1 PATHOLOGY

These lesions are paragangliomas or chemodectomas derived from the neural crest and they are usually benign. A low malignancy rate (3-5%) is recorded. The glomus tumours may be associated with a carotid body tumour or phaechromocytoma. They are found in the lower middle ear (glomus tympanicum) and on the jugular bulb (glomus jugulare).

12.2 PRESENTATION

The history is one of unilateral deafness and pulsatile tinnitus. Vertigo and sensorineural deafness may occur with auditory nerve involvement and nerves VII-XII may be affected by tumour extension in the jugular foramen. On examination, a red mass may be evident behind the lower tympanic membrane, perhaps with a serous effusion. Angiography shows a vascular blush at the site of the lesion. Erosion of the base of the skull may be shown on tomography in larger lesions.

12.3 MANAGEMENT

Smaller lesions (glomus tympanicum) may be removed simply from the middle ear under the operating microscope, but larger masses (glomus jugulare) may require pre-operative embolization under radiological guidance plus external carotid ligation to limit blood loss. Neurosurgical involvement is required in lesions with intracranial extension.

CHAPTER 12:
FACIAL PALSY

INTRODUCTION

Paralysis of the facial nerve, although not a disease of the ear itself, often arises within the ear. These paralyses therefore commonly require the diagnostic skills of the otologist, together with his surgical expertise, for their correction. It is emphasised that many cases of facial palsy are surgical emergencies. Immediate otological assessment is mandatory to achieve optimal cure rates in this group.

1. ANATOMY

The facial nerve has four fibre types:

1.1 MOTOR
1.2 SECRETOMOTOR } Nervus intermedius
1.3 TASTE
1.4 TACTILE (controversial)

1.1 MOTOR

fibres arise in the facial nucleus in the pons and pass unrelayed to the facial muscles.

1.2 SECRETOMOTOR

(parasympathetic) fibres arise from the superior salivary nucleus. Some pass out with the greater superficial petrosal nerve and eventually to the lacrimal gland and nasal mucosa. Other fibres pass in the main trunk to the chorda tympani and thence to the submandibular and sublingual glands.

1.3 TASTE FIBRES,

from the tractus solitarius, relay in the geniculate ganglion and pass:

(a) to the palate

(b) to the anterior two-thirds of the tongue.

1.4 Whether the facial nerve contains cutaneous sensory fibres remains uncertain, but their presence is suspected by the Herpes Zoster Oticus vesicles on the drum, posterior wall of the external auditory meatus and the pinna in the Ramsay-Hunt Syndrome.

2. COURSE OF THE NERVE

The facial nerve leaves the lower edge of the pons in two roots - the motor root and the nervus intermedius. These enter the IAM and merge on their arrival at the geniculate ganglion. The trunk then passes horizontally backwards just above the stapes, then immediately turns vertically downwards to pass out via the stylomastoid foramen. Passing anteriorly and laterally, it then breaks up into the plexus within the parotid, branching over the face. Within this plexus are many interconnecting branches, a feature which is valuable in crossfacial grafting. (Fig. 66)

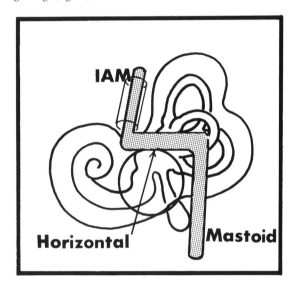

Figure 66. Intratemporal course of the facial nerve. The main trunk and the nervus intermedius are found in the internal auditory meatus (IAM) ending at the geniculate ganglion. The nerve then turns posteriorly and passes horizontally just superior to the oval window. At the postero-inferior end of the lateral semicircular canal the nerve turns inferiorly, passes vertically through the mastoid and passes out through the stylomastoid foramen.

2.1. CLINICALLY IMPORTANT BRANCHES (Fig. 67)

(a) Greater superficial petrosal nerve. Taste and secretomotor fibres to the sphenopalatine ganglion. The secretomotor fibres pass to the lacrimal gland and nasal mucosa, the taste fibres to the palate.

(b) The nerve to the stapedius. Motor fibres innervating the stapedius muscle itself.

(c) Chorda tympani. Taste and secretomotor fibres to the lingual nerve. The taste fibres pass to the anterior two-thirds of the tongue and the secretomotor fibres to the submandibular and sublingual glands.

submandibular and sublingual glands.

(d) Motor branches to the facial muscles.

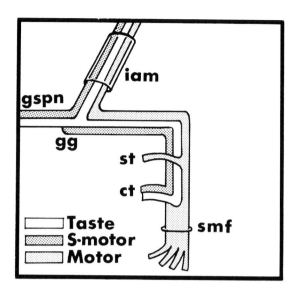

Figure 67. Functional plan of the facial nerve in the temporal bone. iam: internal auditory meatus; gspn: greater superficial petrosal nerve; gg: geniculate ganglion; st: nerve to stapedius; ct: chorda tympani; smf: stylomastoid foramen.

3. AETIOLOGY

Facial palsy may arise from upper or lower motor neurone lesions. In cases of upper motor neurone lesions, due to CNS fibre crossover the upper part of the face remains at least partially mobile during emotional expression. Frequently therefore, upper motor neurone lesions can be differentiated clinically. Upper motor neurone lesions can be due to a wide range of CNS pathology which is beyond the scope of this work.

3.1 AETIOLOGY OF LOWER MOTOR NEURONE PARALYSIS

3.1.1 IDIOPATHIC - "BELLS PALSY"

3.1.2 TRAUMA:

(a) Fractures

(b) External trauma

(c) Surgical

3.1.3 INFECTIONS:

(a) Acute otitis media

(b) Chronic otitis media

(c) Cholesteatoma

(d) Herpes Zoster Oticus

3.1.4 ACOUSTIC NEUROMA, OTHER INTRACRANIAL MASSES

3.1.5 MISCELLANEOUS, EG. COLLAGEN DISEASE, POLYNEURITIS.

4. HISTORY

The patient is questioned on the duration of the palsy, how rapidly it developed, and whether any causative or associated symptoms were present. Particular reference is made to the cardinal ear symptoms (pain, discharge, deafness, tinnitus and vertigo). The presence of any CNS symptoms is sought, with emphasis on posterior fossa or cerebellar signs.)

5. EXAMINATION

The palsy itself is assessed to ascertain whether the lesion is of an upper or lower motor neurone type by assessing emotional or involuntary facial movement. Care is taken to fully assess and note the extent of the paralysis in each of the areas supplied, in order to assess progress later. In complete cases, sagging of the face at rest due to loss of muscle tone may be noted, particularly in the elderly.

Accurate assessment of the ear is essential. Due to wax in the external meatus, subtle changes in the tympanic membrane, or a curved canal, causative ear diseases may be difficult to diagnose. An early otologist's opinion regarding the ear's condition is desirable to detect a curable lesion which requires prompt treatment. The CNS is fully assessed with emphasis on the cerebellum and the cranial nerves V-XII.

Extratemporal causes in the parotid, upper neck and face are excluded, and a check is made for the vesicles of Herpes Zoster on the EAM and pinna.

5.1 ASSESSMENT OF THE LEVEL OF BLOCK

Several tests are available to help localise the lesion in lower motor neurone lesions:

5.1.1 SCHIRMER'S TEST.

Lesions at the level of the geniculate ganglion or above reduce lacrimation in the ipsilateral eye. To assess this loss, lacrimation is stimulated and measured on 5mm absorbent paper strips hooked over and hanging from the lower eyelid. The test is positive if the affected side exhibits markedly less lacrimation than the normal. (Fig. 68)

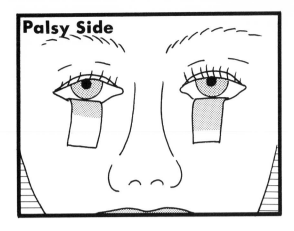

Figure 66. Schirmer's test. Litmus paper is hooked onto the lower eyelids and lacrimation is stimulated. If a facial palsy at the geniculate ganglion or above is present, lacrimation will be significantly depressed on the palsy side

5.1.2 STAPEDIUS REFLEX

The presence or absence of this reflex is assessed with impedance audiometry. If Schirmer's test is negative and there is no stapedius reflex, then the lesion lies on the horizontal segment of the facial nerve, ie. between the geniculate ganglion and the nerve to the stapedius.

5.1.3 TASTE TESTING, ELECTROGUSTOMETRY

Testing of the taste with chemicals (salt, sugar, etc.) or electrically will show if the lesion is above or below the origin of the chorda tympani. The gustometer produces a sour or metallic sensation on stimulation via an electrode on the tongue. If the taste is intact, the lesion lies further down the vertical segment of the facial nerve or is extratemporal.

5.2 TESTS OF MOTOR FUNCTION

In cases of partial function, the nerve trunk is necessarily intact and electrodiagnostic tests have limited value. In complete palsy, however, they are of considerable prognostic help. Three main techniques are used:

5.2.1 NERVE EXCITABILITY TEST
5.2.2 ELECTROMYOGRAPHY
5.2.3 ELECTRONEURONOGRAPHY

5.2.1 NERVE EXCITABILITY TEST.

The nerve is stimulated by an electrode on the skin over the stylomastoid foramen and the smallest current intensity required to produce facial movement is compared with that for the normal side. The difference should only be 3-10mA and greater differences indicate axon degeneration rather than neuropraxia.

5.2.2 ELECTROMYOGRAPHY

This is performed using a needle electrode inserted into the facial muscle. Several types of muscle activity can be recorded:

(a) Volitional motor potentials. If a clinically completely paralysed muscle produces muscle action potentials on attempts at voluntary movement, it can be concluded that subclinical voluntary action is present and that nerve continuity remains intact.

(b) Denervation potentials or fibrillation potentials occur with axon degeneration but appear only about ten days after the onset of palsy. Their absence for some weeks after the palsy may point to a better prognosis.

(c) Polyphasic motor unit potentials. These patterns appear during re-innervation of muscle whose motor supply has degenerated. In facial palsies they appear about $2\frac{1}{2}$-3 months after the palsy first appears.

5.2.3 ELECTRONEURONOGRAPHY (ENoG)

This test provides the best quantitative assessment of nerve function and is valuable in assessing clinical progress of degeneration after a complete palsy. A bipolar electrode stimulates the facial trunk just anterior to the mastoid and action potentials are read by an electrode over the nasolabial fold. The affected and non-affected sides are compared; degeneration is detected by diminishing potentials on successive tests.

6. CLINICAL CONDITIONS

6.1 BELLS PALSY

Bells Palsy refers to those facial palsies for which no identifiable cause can be found. Some are thought to be viral in origin and minor epidemics may occur.

6.1.1 PATHOLOGY

Only scanty histological data is available, showing non-specific hyperaemia and axon degeneration. Surgeons decompressing the nerve for this condition note considerable oedema and increased vascularity.

6.1.2 PRESENTATION

The palsy is not associated with causative symptoms. Pain is felt in some cases, and taste aberrations or phonophobia may be present due to a chorda block or a stapedius paralysis. The ipsilateral eye may water or ache due to desiccation. There is a tendency to recurrence of the condition in individuals who have suffered a previous episode. Examination shows total or partial lower motor neurone paralysis. The CNS, ear, and extratemporal areas are normal. Particular care is taken to exclude the presence of herpes vesicles.

6.1.3 INVESTIGATION

Radiology excludes intratemporal or intracranial lesions. The level of the block is located using the Schirmer's, stapedial reflex, and taste tests. Electrodiagnostic tests confirm complete or partial paralysis and later indicate if degeneration has occurred.

6.1.4 PROGNOSIS

Four clinical features aid in assessing the patient's outlook:

(a) Age - As a rule, the elderly fare worse than the young.

(b) Speed of onset - Rapid deterioration of function is more ominous than slow progression over several days.

(c) Complete paralysis carries a worse prognosis.

(d) Pain with the onset of the palsy is felt to indicate a poorer prognosis.

Seventy to eighty per cent of cases obtain excellent recovery, 10% have a good recovery, but 10% achieve poor or no recovery.

6.1.5 MANAGEMENT

Urgent assessment is desirable, particularly to exclude reversible otological conditions. The condition of each branch should be assessed and described at the first presentation, for later review. Incomplete palsies may be observed carefully without intervention, but the patient is warned to notify any deterioration.

(a) Medical Management
In palsies with a clinically better prognosis, steroid therapy is commenced after checking for contra-indications to these drugs. Prednisone, 25mg q.i.d. for five days, is given followed by a reducing programme thereafter.

(b) Surgical Decompression
In a select group of cases in whom the prognosis is poor but who present within a few hours of the onset, consideration can be given to surgical decompression of the nerve within the temporal bone. This is done to alleviate the pressure of oedema and to permit optimal recovery conditions. The approach depends on the site of the lesion. The procedure requires high skills and is not without risk to the patient's hearing.

(c) Other
In established complete palsies, lateral tarsorrhaphy may be required to prevent corneal ulceration. Plastic sling procedures to lift sagging facial tissues may help cosmetically. Cross-facial grafting is performed using a cutaneous nerve graft from the leg to transmit impulses from one plexus to the other. In skilled hands this may obtain pleasing symmetry of facial expression.

6.2 TRAUMATIC PALSIES

Division of the nerve by trauma or surgery requires exploration and possibly grafting if division is complete, or decompression and re-approximation if not.

6.3 INFECTION

Palsies due to middle ear infection occur with or without cholesteatoma. The presence of the latter is an indication for urgent surgery to remove the infected sac from the middle ear. In cases of acute otitis media, a myringotomy is performed for drainage, and a vent tube is inserted. If mastoiditis is present, a cortical mastoidectomy is performed. Serial cleaning by suction toilet under the operating microscope is performed. Gentamicin ear drops and high dosage antibiotics (as for acute otitis media) are employed to clear the infection as rapidly as possible. Systemic gentamicin and ciprofloxacin are used if a palsy results from chronic otitis media or cholesteatoma.

6.4 HERPES ZOSTER OTICUS

The Ramsay-Hunt Syndrome consists of facial paralysis, herpes zoster vesicles on the external auditory meatus and pinna, and labyrinthine dysfunction, often severe. The pathology is that of diffuse facial nerve inflammation (not only the geniculate ganglion) plus diffuse cochlear, vestibular and auditory nerve lesions. Clinically the patient suffers from the above features with pain preceding the vesicle formation. Vesicles over other nerve areas may be present in the pharynx, head and neck, or trunk.

Management is by general support plus early steroid therapy to preserve hearing. The outlook is poorer than for Bells Palsy.

6.5 INTRATEMPORAL OR POSTERIOR FOSSA SPACE OCCUPYING LESION

Facial palsy complicating these conditions requires urgent exploration. Salvage of the nerve may be difficult due to gross displacement or splaying of the nerve fibres.

Pure tone audiometry (PTA) is a simple and accurate method of assessing hearing. Many conditions produce characteristic pure tone patterns which may permit rapid clinical evaluation. The figures below provide a synopsis of classical audiograms which are frequently encountered in clinical practice.

Right Air Conduction: o-o-o
Left Air Conduction: x-x-x
Right Bone Conduction: [—[—[
Left Bone Conduction:]—]—]

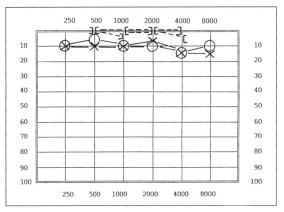

Figure 1. Normal pure tone audiogram performed in soundproof conditions. Levels down to 5 to 10 decibels may be encountered in children, 5 to 15 in adults. There is minimal difference between air and bone levels.

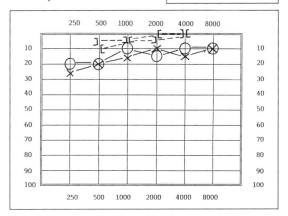

Figure 2. Normal PTA, imperfect testing conditions. Mild low frequency losses are common when soundproofed conditions are suboptimal. Other mild losses are common in field testing, due to instrument calibration variation, staff training, distractions, and other difficulties.

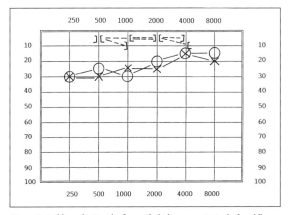

Figure 3. Mild conductive deafness. Slight losses are typical of middle ear effusions, recent infection, minor past middle ear disease, or mild drum collapse.

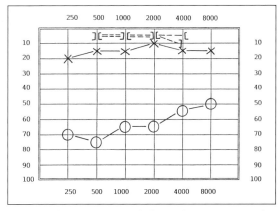

Figure 4. Substantial conductive deafness, right ear. Major external or middle ear disease such as congenital deformities may produce losses up to 70–80 decibels if the cochlea is normal.

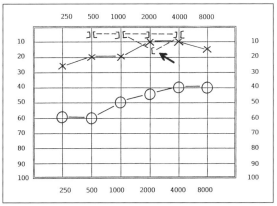

Figure 5. Otosclerosis. This common fixation of the stapes footplate produces a conductive loss, usually maximal in the lower frequencies. Typically, a slight depression in the bone conduction levels is seen at 2000 cycles per second—a "Carhart's notch" carried.

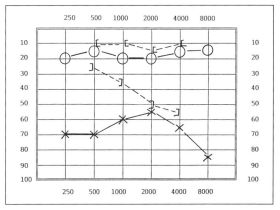

Figure 6. Mixed deafness (combined conductive and sensorineural). Combined conductive (usually low frequency) and sensorineural (usually high frequency) losses are commonly found in otosclerosis or long-standing chronic otitis media.

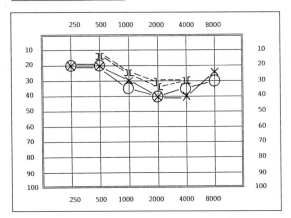

Figure 7. Right sensorineural deafness. Unilateral losses of this extent in an adult are frequently due to viral or microvascular origins, but a thorough assessment of these cases to exclude acoustic neuroma is mandatory. Childhood cases are usually congenital or secondary to measles, mumps, or other viruses.

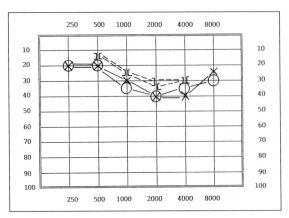

Figure 8. Congenital sensorineural deafness. Bilateral mid-frequency "cookie-bite" pattern nerve losses are genetically determined and may be progressive. Follow up is required to check for the latter.

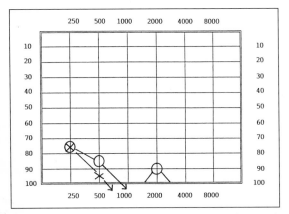

Figure 9. Profound bilateral sensorineural losses. In an infant, speech development would be unlikely without the use of a cochlear implant. The advent of these implants has given a new life to many previously severely deaf individuals.

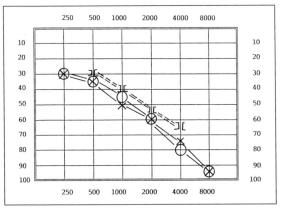

Figure 10. Presbyacusis. Symmetrical, bilateral sloping high frequency nerve losses are typical of the effects of age. Hearing aids may help, but the sufferer frequently complains of speech discrimination difficulties, particularly in noisy conditions, due to the loss of much of the consonant content of speech.

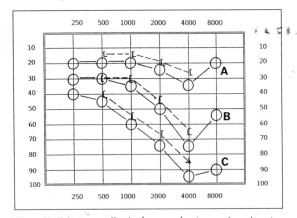

*Figure 11. Noise trauma. Hearing loss secondary to excessive noise exposure initially presents as a mild nerve loss at 4000 cycles per second **A**. Further exposure results in progressive high frequency loss **B**. Prolonged severe damage gives PTA patterns similar to advanced presbyacusis, as the 4000 cps depression is gradually lost (**C**).*

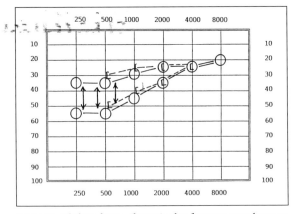

Figure 12. Ménière's disease. Fluctuating low frequency nerve losses are typical of the fully established clinical presentation of endolymphatic hydrops. Similar patterns may be found in tertiary syphilis or some autoimmune conditions.